STAN,

Continue to be
a light in dark
places. Your spirit
is needed as our
country heals.
Much love
my dear brother!!!

Bobby
King
CLA 25

UNDERTHESKIN

ALSO BY LINDA VILLAROSA

Passing for Black
Body & Soul

UNDERTHESKIN

THE HIDDEN TOLL OF RACISM ON AMERICAN LIVES AND ON THE HEALTH OF OUR NATION

LINDA VILLAROSA

DOUBLEDAY   NEW YORK

All rights reserved. Published in the United States by Doubleday, a
division of Penguin Random House LLC, New York, and distributed in
Canada by Penguin Random House Canada Limited, Toronto.

www.doubleday.com

DOUBLEDAY and the portrayal of an anchor with a dolphin are
registered trademarks of Penguin Random House LLC.

Grateful acknowledgment is made to She Writes Press for permission to reprint
excerpts of poems from *Soul Psalms* by U-Meleni Mhlaba-Adebo. Reprinted
by permission of She Writes Press, a division of SparkPoint Studio, LLC.

Book design by Michael Collica
Jacket art by Sean Gerard Clark
Jacket design by Emily Mahon

Library of Congress Cataloging-in-Publication Data
Names: Villarosa, Linda, author.
Title: Under the skin: the hidden toll of racism on American
lives and on the health of our nation / Linda Villarosa.
Description: First edition. | New York : Doubleday, [2022] | Includes index.
Identifiers: LCCN 2021043388 (print) | LCCN 2021043389 (ebook) |
ISBN 9780385544887 (hardcover) | ISBN 9780385544894 (ebook)
Subjects: LCSH: African Americans—Health and hygiene—United
States. | Discrimination in medical care—United States. | Racism in
medicine—United States. | African Americans—Social conditions.
Classification: LCC RA448.5.N4 V55 2022 (print) |
LCC RA448.5.N4 (ebook) | DDC 362.1089/96073—dc23
LC record available at https://lccn.loc.gov/2021043388
LC ebook record available at https://lccn.loc.gov/2021043389

MANUFACTURED IN THE UNITED STATES OF AMERICA

1 3 5 7 9 10 8 6 4 2

First Edition

To my parents, Andres and Clara Villarosa, with gratitude

Underneath my skin

There are layers of pain
Simmering endlessly
Every day
I am seconds away from cracking

—"Breaking Point," U-Meleni Mhlaba-Adebo

CONTENTS

UNDERTHESKIN

EVERYTHING I THOUGHT WAS WRONG

Although the United States has the most advanced medical technology in the world—and spends more on health care than anywhere else—we lag behind all other wealthy nations in key measures of health that serve as a proxy for our overall well-being. It starts at birth and ends with death. The United States has the highest rate of infant mortality and the lowest life expectancy in comparison with other wealthy countries. An American woman is more likely to die as a result of pregnancy and childbirth than women in other countries of comparable wealth. That rate is higher now than it was in the 1990s, even though most of these deaths of mothers are avoidable.

The poor health outcomes of the world's wealthiest nation are often presented as a mystery, yet their root causes are hiding in plain sight: these disparities are driven by inequality and discrimination, which lead to poor health in people of color in the United States, particularly African Americans. The health outcomes of Black Americans are by several measures on par with people living in far poorer nations. At every stage of life, Blacks have poorer health outcomes than whites and, in most cases, than other ethnic groups. Black babies are more than twice as likely as white babies to die at birth or in the first year of life—a racial gap that adds up to thousands of lost lives every year. Blacks in every age-group under sixty-five have significantly higher death rates than whites. Black life expectancy at birth is several years lower than that of whites. African Americans have elevated death rates from conditions such as diabetes, stroke, and heart disease that among whites are found more commonly at older ages. In a phrase, African Americans "live sicker and die quicker," which, if you estimate years of life lost because of deaths that could've been prevented, adds up to tens of thousands of lost years.

Too often this story of inequity and disadvantage in health gets dismissed as "only" affecting the poor, or being one of class, not race. It is indisputable that poverty creates emotional disruption, inequality, and fear. Health-care facilities in lower-income communities are often underfunded and left to waste away. The poorest communities lack access to healthy food, clean water and air, and outdoor space—as well as jobs, safe living conditions, and quality education. This in itself is unfair and tragic and affects people of all races and ethnicities who live in pockets of rural, urban, and suburban poverty across the country. Too frequently, rather than taking into account these structural inequities, we blame the individuals, by insisting they wouldn't be poor if they worked harder and wouldn't be sick if they were educated and simply took better care of themselves.

However, poverty is not the sole factor in who gets sick and who doesn't, in who survives and who passes away; it just makes the situation that much worse. Even when income, education, and access to health care are matched, African Americans remain disadvantaged and racial disparities in health cut lives short. College-educated Black mothers, for example, are more likely to die, almost die, or lose their babies than white mothers who haven't finished high school.

I am a Black American and have been a journalist and author in both ethnic and mainstream media for several decades. Most of my work has looked at the health of African Americans, particularly Black women, and at racial health disparities. Of course, I have long understood that *something* about being Black has led to the documented poor health of Black Americans. But in recent years I have come to understand that much of what I believed about health disparities and inequality in the United States was wrong. The *something* that is making Black Americans sicker is not race per se, or the lack of money, education, information, and access to health services that can be tied to being Black in America. It is also not genes or something inherently wrong or inferior about the Black body. The *something* is racism. Income, education, determination, and self-empowerment can help individual Black Americans but cannot entirely erase the negative effects of centuries of discrimination, and ongoing bias, on the health of African Americans. To put it in the plainest terms, from birth to death the impact on the bodies of Black Americans of living in communities that have been harmed by long-standing racial discrimination, of a deeply rooted and dangerous racial bias in our health-care system, and of the insidious consequences of present-day racism affects who lives and who dies. These factors create physical vulnerability and systemic disadvantages that education, income, and access to health care cannot erase. This inequality, born more than four hundred years ago and embedded in every structure and institution of American society, including the health-care system, is driving our country's poor national health outcomes relative to the rest of the developed world. It has taken me three decades of reporting on the health of African Americans and several disturbing personal medical crises to understand the ways discrimination and bias contribute to poor health outcomes primarily in African Americans, but in reality in all oppressed people.

In the mid-1980s, I became a contributing nutrition and fitness writer for *Essence* magazine, and eventually the publication's health editor. Like so many other Black women before and after me, I remember seeing *Essence* at my grandmother's bedside and on my mother's coffee table when I was growing up. It was first published in 1970, during the intersection of the Black Power and women's liberation movements and served as a bible for Black women. The mission, instilled in everyone on the staff by our editor in chief, Susan L. Taylor, was clear: in a world full of negative representation and damaging mythology, give Black women positive images of themselves and empower what would eventually grow from fifty thousand to more than one million readers and a reach of more than eight million subscribers with information about relationships, finances, careers, travel, family, spirituality, food, health, and, most important, self-love and acceptance, to make their lives better.

At *Essence,* my personal mission was unambiguous: fix the health crisis in Black America. At the time, from the late 1980s to the end of the last millennium, I understood that Black America was experiencing a life-crushing constellation of health problems; Black people were contracting serious illnesses at younger ages than other Americans and living fewer years. I was sure, as so many others believed then and still believe today, that poverty was solely to blame. In 1985, I was transfixed by the Heckler Report, issued by the U.S. Department of Health and Human Services (HHS) and released that October, which took a research deep dive into racial health disparities. The ground-shattering document was pulled together by a nineteen-member task force of senior scientists and officials at HHS who analyzed existing data about race, death, and disease in the United States. They examined the underlying factors and consulted with experts outside the government who specialized in the health of people of color. This publication marked the first time the government had comprehensively studied the health status of people of color, and it elevated the issue of health inequality to the national stage. I ordered a print copy of the 239-page study and read it like a novel.

Named for the HHS secretary at the time, Margaret Heckler, the report estimated that there were more than eighteen thousand "excess deaths" each year among Blacks because of heart disease and stroke, compared with the number of deaths that would occur if their health was on par with that of whites. It also pointed to 8,116 excess deaths from cancer, 6,178 from infant mortality, and 1,850 from diabetes. It made me ache to consider the thousands of Black men, women, and babies dead every year from medical problems we knew how to prevent and treat. Heckler, a pro-life Reagan Republican, called this shameful inequality "an affront both to our ideals and to the ongoing genius of American medicine."

The Heckler Report recommended no new government funding to attack the crisis. The report did discuss what we now call the "social determinants of health," conditions like poor housing, crime, pollution, shortage of healthy food, and lack of medical services that affect mental and physical health. But it neglected to mention the Reagan administration's cutting or freezing federal dollars for Medicaid, food stamps, family planning, and other supportive services, which would make health disparities grow, not shrink. Heckler insisted that "money was not the answer." There was no mention of discrimination and bias either inside or outside the medical-care system. Instead, the report advised Black Americans to save themselves by improving their health through education, self-help, and self-care. The government's role was to bolster data collection and communication between agencies and expand health education. Heckler lay the blame bluntly at a press conference following the release of the report: "Progress depends more on education and a change in personal behavior than it does on more doctors, more hospitals, or more technology."

Within this largely well-meaning report lurked the assumption that Black people, individually and collectively, were irresponsible, careless, uneducated, and making thoughtless choices that led to this health crisis in the first place. Edith Irby Jones, MD, then the president of the National Medical Association, the professional organization for Black physicians, called out Heckler on this point in a 1986 essay in her group's journal. Dr. Jones wrote that Heckler's "implication, of course, is that if Black people would only 'behave' their health problems would be solved . . . Well, as Black Americans we know it is not as simple as that. Blaming the patient will not cure the ills of America's underserved minorities." She also recommended "*hope* in place of hopelessness, *service* in place of self-serving moralizing."

At the time, I didn't question the report. I was excited to see a document full of evidence of racial health disparities, developed by experts and blessed by the federal government, and used it as a mandate, firmly believing that if we—Black Americans—know better, we do better. The report also dovetailed perfectly with my own belief in self-help and the mandate of the magazine. I approached *Essence's* mission with passion and steely focus, through a Washingtonian (Booker T.) lens of individual self-improvement—helping people help themselves and uplifting those who couldn't. I never strayed from the belief that people had the power to save their own lives in the face of the health disparities described in detail in the Heckler Report. I understood that my life's work at the time was to provide our readers with solid, practical self-help information about diet, exercise, and other kinds of self-care so individuals could be healthier, which would raise the health status of the entire Black community. I imagined a kind of trickle-down effect from the health information our magazine provided: I promoted an each-one-teach-one mentality that encouraged readers to make sure all the "sisters" in the lives of our largely middle-class audience (read: your less educated and privileged friends and family) understood the importance of good health and how to achieve it. It was us and them—us, the educated middle-class Blacks like me and my relatives, and them, the economically challenged Blacks whose image shone brightly in full-spectrum dysfunction in the American media, then as now dominated by upper-middle-class, largely white male producers, editors, reporters, and writers. At *Essence,* our staff of mainly Black women did not just feel responsible for those less fortunate Blacks; we were actually tasked with saving them. I recall being in an *Essence* staff meeting where our editor explained that each of us was responsible for the lives of eight Black women. I remember coming home late one night, and as I was walking up the subway steps, exhausted on my way back to Brooklyn from Manhattan, I thought, "No wonder I'm so tired. I've got eight women tethered to me, and I just dragged them up the stairs!"

The Heckler Report's conclusions also fit comfortably with what I'm ashamed to admit were my own narrow views of Black communities in America. While I wasn't crass enough to blame poor African Americans for their plight, I fell prey to limiting, media-driven stereotypes of Black people. I had spent my early years growing up on the South Side of Chicago in the all-Black neighborhood near where my mother had been born and raised, and we lived in a building my grandparents owned. As a child, I was influenced by my parents' complaints about Chicago and whisper-hiss conversations about how they needed to *get out* of the city and start their own life. By the time I was in third grade, the city's homicide rate had more than doubled from a decade before, and nearly a third of all Black residents lived below the poverty level. At first, my parents wanted to move to a predominantly white suburb near my father's job as a bacteriologist at Edward Hines Jr. VA Hospital. But while looking for a home, my mother asked a police officer if the area would be safe for a Black family, and he told her, "I can't guarantee that we could protect you and your family." Finally, in 1969, my father requested a transfer to Denver, and my parents packed up our Rambler station wagon and moved the family to the suburb of Lakewood, Colorado. We were part of a larger trend of Black suburbanization that began to reverse the tendency of Chocolate Cities and Vanilla Suburbs. In the 1970s, the overall Black population in American suburbs increased by 70 percent as African American families like mine moved to the suburbs, taking advantage of a world newly expanded by civil rights legislation that finally dislodged some of the institutional discrimination in housing and education. Leaving Chicago, the only city she had ever known, and moving far away from her parents and extended family, was gut-wrenching for my mother. But like so many Black parents of the era, mine wanted to get out of the hood and give my sister and me a better childhood than they had had. To them that meant we would grow up in a house with a backyard, not an apartment near the Dan Ryan Expressway, and go to a school with a cafeteria, not run to the church across the street at noon to eat a free lunch served by Christian volunteers in the basement. We would learn alongside the white kids, play outside with them in the safe streets of our suburban community, and get all of

the privileges generally reserved for them. We were what are sometimes called Integration Babies.

The year after Martin Luther King Jr. was assassinated, as we drove
up to our new ranch house just west of Denver—so much larger
than the apartment where we had lived with my grandparents in
Chicago—I asked, "Daddy, do we have to share it with another family?" My little sister was even more amazed: "Are we rich?" Then we
saw it. Somebody had written "Niggers Get Out" on the garage door
and on the pavement on the driveway. Some of the neighbors—all
white—were trying to scrub off the words before we arrived. But it
was too late. My father wanted to get right back in the car and drive
home to Chicago, but my mother—and the neighbors—persuaded
him to stay. We later found out it had been the twin boys two houses
down who delivered the newspaper who had defiled our new home
on a dare. Their father made them apologize and deliver the paper
for two months for free, paid out of their allowance, as punishment.

A few days later, when I started third grade, no one spoke to me
at all for two weeks. I later learned that the principal had called a
school-wide assembly the Friday before I arrived to explain to my
classmates that Alameda Elementary was getting its first Black students. The other third graders were so afraid of saying the wrong
thing that they said nothing at all. Finally, months later, a little girl
with large brown eyes, freckles, and pigtails asked if she could walk
home from school with me. I exhaled, and she became my first
friend. I worked hard to hold on to my white friends. Like many of
us who grew up in predominantly white spaces, I understood that I
needed to be twice as good as everyone else to receive half as much
respect, and I became the poster girl for overachievement. In high
school, I earned nearly straight As, was captain of the track team,
an editor of the yearbook, and president of my class. What I would
later understand as high-effort coping never prevented me from feeling like a fly in the buttermilk, but it did allow me to find a place.
Fitting in demanded a kind of Stockholm syndrome trade-off: it
meant absorbing the stereotypes about Black people and communi-

ties, pervasive in every corner of American culture, that most white people accept as truth. To reconcile these images with my reality, I had to believe my family and I were exceptions, an idea thoroughly endorsed by others. I can no longer recall how many times people said to me, "You don't seem Black," or "You aren't like other Black people."

I would not have a true understanding of the breadth and depth of structural racism for another few decades, when I became a college professor and had to first learn about, then teach, a version of critical race theory to my Black studies students. Without a more sophisticated racial justice framework, our family members lived by a pieced-together set of principles that included hard work, determination, education, and religious conviction that we believed made us better Blacks, the good Negroes. While this philosophy improved our lives, it was not the full picture.

I was most influenced by the story of my grandparents, who each managed to flee the limited opportunities and racial terrorism of the South and get out of two different cities in Mississippi during the Great Migration in the late 1920s to land in the South Side of Chicago. My grandmother was particularly inspiring. She left Iuka, Mississippi, following her seven siblings, and most of this extended family settled on or near South Vernon Avenue, where they created a kind of warm, familiar Mississippi cocoon, relying on each other for comfort and support. They bought their homes and, in my grandparents' case, buildings, got educated, and launched businesses and careers, overcoming what I believed were only personal challenges. I was proud of my grandparents, inspired by our family lore of individual grit and success. My family judged those who either didn't get out of the South or didn't find success in the North as less smart, motivated, and hardworking. Later, after my immediate family moved out of Chicago, my mother, father, sister, and I created a walled-off microcosm of four in Denver so that we were able to at first merely survive living in an all-white community and eventually actually thrive. We believed Black people like my family had the responsibility to give back to those who had less ingenuity, education, money, and work ethic, because that was the price of success, Black success.

About five years after I became health editor of *Essence*—and after writing and editing a whole lot of articles with advice about "self-health"—I would begin to understand that those less fortunate sisters and brothers of my experience and imagination were not to blame for the health disparities that plagued Black America and being middle class didn't entirely protect any of the good Negroes. In other words, I got an early inkling that though being poor matters greatly where health is concerned, race, even in the absence of poverty, matters too. Something began to shift when I met Harold Freeman, MD, the director of surgery at Harlem Hospital who had recently served as the national president of the American Cancer Society. He had co-written a groundbreaking article, "Excess Mortality in Harlem," published in the January 1990 issue of *The New England Journal of Medicine*. The piece explained that even as life expectancy was rising in the United States for people of all races, Black men in Harlem lived fewer years than their counterparts in the impoverished country of Bangladesh. This framing put racial health disparities into sharp focus, and the article received widespread media attention.

Like most readers, I was shocked by this dire situation, which I still understood as affecting only poor Black people who lived in impoverished communities, lacked access to health care, and either didn't understand how to take care of themselves or were unable to because of their economic circumstances. In those days, Harlem was scarred by an epidemic of crack, violence, and HIV/AIDS. In the neighborhood—at the time, still majority Black as it had been since its sparkling Renaissance days at the beginning of the twentieth century—40 percent of families lived below the government-defined poverty line, and the death rate from homicide had quadrupled in the previous twenty years. Neither the city, state, nor national government offered a real lifeline.

I met Dr. Freeman in 1991 when he came to Harvard to talk to my fellowship program about his *New England Journal of Medicine* article. With calm deliberation, this tall, elegant physician disrupted my vision of Harlem and other Black communities throughout the United States. He detailed a cascade of health conditions triggered by inadequate facilities, lack of access to health insurance, and a shortage of medical personnel, healthy food, safe neighborhoods, and basic education. He called the problem a national tragedy, an emergency analogous to a hurricane, flood, or other ruinous natural disaster, yet one for which no one was sounding the alarm. Afterward, I introduced myself and asked him to confirm what I thought I knew: that the issues he described were strictly a result of poverty. But Dr. Freeman took me aside and patiently corrected my thinking. Yes, being poor mattered, because poverty is synonymous with lack of education, inadequate housing, insufficient nutrition, barriers to medical services, and focus on day-to-day survival rather than long-term and preventive care. But he also pointed out that the image of Harlem in the popular imagination as a broken-down, crime-riddled battleground was incomplete. In fact, he said, Harlem was economically diverse—much like my neighborhood in Chicago—with a quarter of the community comprising middle- to upper-class African Americans, like my grandparents and great-aunts and great-uncles.

He looked me straight in the eye and said, "If you really care about these issues and want to make a difference, you must *not* use race as a proxy for poverty or poverty as a proxy for race. They intersect and overlap, but to really understand the health of this country, you have to be more sophisticated than assuming that only poor Blacks are affected by this crisis. Look deeper, think differently." He warned me that many scientists and researchers conflate race and class, under the assumption that all Black people are poor, and all poor people are Black. "Don't let that be a blind spot," he told me.

By the end of the event, he had agreed to allow me to spend the day with him at Harlem Hospital to see where and how he worked and to listen to his patients to get a deeper understanding of the issues.

On the day I was to shadow him, I followed Dr. Freeman down the corridor to his office, looking like a very quiet medical student. I teared up, struck by how he looked like my father in so many ways, down to his long-legged, wide-stride gait, spit-shined shoes, his back slightly rounded in the way of tall, kind men. At the end of that day, I couldn't shake the image of one of his patients. She was a well-dressed, professional woman, a soft-spoken single mother in her forties who lived in Harlem and worked as an administrator in a Manhattan office. Her appointment was in the late afternoon, because she was nervous about leaving her job early. She had come to see Dr. Freeman because her breast was "bothering" her. When she lowered her gown, it was obvious what was wrong: she had a large lump on her left breast, darkened like a bruise, pushing through the skin, and painful to the touch. As he examined her, Dr. Freeman asked her gently, without a shred of judgment, only concern, why she hadn't come to see him sooner, when treatment might have made a difference. Her answer surprised me: she hadn't avoided addressing this obvious issue out of ignorance or lack of access to health care, the standard explanations for the racial disparities that plague African Americans in Black communities. This woman had health insurance and access to Dr. Freeman, one of the world's most renowned cancer specialists and a caring Black physician who chose to practice in Harlem. "I was afraid," she said, very slowly, looking down. She paused, before continuing. "I was afraid that if this was serious, I would die and there would be no one to take care of my son." And then she began to cry.

Later, Dr. Freeman told me that she had advanced breast cancer and that she probably wouldn't survive to see her son's next birthday. In her eyes I saw a tragedy that was much more complicated than a Black single mother in Harlem who was dying of breast cancer. Instead, I was able to see, in the body of one woman, several of the complicated themes I would later examine in my work: fear and avoidance of the health-care system, stress, the precariousness of the Black middle class, and the thoughtful heroism of individual provider/researchers like Dr. Freeman. With these concepts in mind, he had founded the Harold P. Freeman Patient Navigation Institute in Harlem to help eliminate barriers to supportive medical care that intersect with race and discrimination and transcend class. Though his insights didn't budge my commitment to self-help advice, Dr. Freeman helped open my mind to a new understanding of the origins of the Black health crisis.

Beginning in the 1990s—the era of the Human Genome Project—scientific research began to drift in the direction of a genetic explanation for Black health problems. If serious diseases were more common among all Black Americans, not just those who were poor and thought to be doing something wrong, then it stood to reason that these health problems could be inherited. In other words, something about being Black was bad for health. In the Black community, most of us had heard of the slavery hypothesis, formed by the hypertension researcher Clarence Grim and others, to explain why African Americans had long had much higher rates of hypertension compared with all other races in the country, and among the highest in the world. This theory was so widespread that as late as 2007, when Mehmet Oz, MD, on *The Oprah Winfrey Show,* asked the talk show host why Blacks have hypertension, Oprah told her audience, "African Americans who survived [the slave trade] were those who could hold more salt in their bodies." Dr. Oz, a physician, replied, "That's perfect." As the theory goes, enslaved Africans who endured the grueling Middle Passage to America had a genetic predisposition to retaining sodium. That is why, while others died of dehydration, they lived to bequeath the gene to their descendants, where it wreaks havoc with their blood pressure. According to the American Heart Association's *current* website, in the section on African Americans, "In people who have this gene, as little as one extra gram (half a teaspoon) of salt could raise blood pressure as much as 5 mm Hg."

For decades, all of the mainstream health organizations and government agencies warned American Blacks specifically to cut down on salt at all costs. Of course, limiting sodium intake is sound advice, and our family followed it to extremes. In my childhood home, when my father was diagnosed with high blood pressure, salt became the enemy—"It will kill Dad," we were told. To this day, everyone reaches for the saltshaker when I cook, because I am still in the habit of under-seasoning food. At *Essence,* we treated salt like crack cocaine; I can't remember how many times I wrote or edited in the words "put down the saltshaker." We stripped recipes of salt, substituting lemon juice, herbs, onion, garlic, and non-salt substitutes to lower sodium content, accompanied articles on hypertension with illustrations of menacing saltshakers, celebrated readers who had made the transition to low-salt diets, and highlighted the cottage industry of cookbooks that explained how to make traditional soul food more healthy by cutting down on salt, fat, and sugar.

Nothing is wrong with reducing salt, avoiding processed food, and finding creative ways to season foods, especially for African Americans, given our high rates of cardiovascular disease. However, at its core, the genetic explanation for those rates lacks evidence. In fact, no data proves that salt-depleting illnesses like dehydration and diarrhea were responsible for a significant number of deaths on slave ships. Instead, countless studies show that along with a diet high in salt and fat, being overweight and a lack of exercise can raise blood pressure. Less discussed, often ignored, but also proven is the link between hypertension and stressful environments and situations, including living with bias and discrimination. Though genetic explanations for poor Black health outcomes have been disproven, they linger in medical education and practice and in the media.

At *Essence,* I operated under the firm belief that Black people weren't paying attention to health information or making positive lifestyle changes because the information was dry, complicated, poorly packaged and explained, and culturally tone-deaf, and to be honest, much of it was. The solution then was "self-health" information packaged specifically for African Americans and presented in a "culturally competent" way—a buzz phrase popular in health and medical circles. If individual Black people could understand how to take care of themselves, and their families, the health crisis would be solved.

In 1992, I signed a contract with HarperCollins to write *Body &*

Soul: The Black Women's Guide to Physical Health and Emotional Well-Being, which I pitched as a kind of *Our Bodies, Ourselves*–style self-help manual for Black women. It would include topics covered by mainstream health books, including nutrition, fitness, sex, sexuality, pregnancy, parenting, and aging, but from a unique Afrocentric perspective. It also discussed more serious topics such as abortion, domestic violence, HIV/AIDS, sexual abuse, and workplace discrimination, mainly through my self-health lens. In meetings with publishers who asked, "Why do Black women need their own health book?" I answered, "Because we don't see ourselves in other health and wellness books." I asked them to consider what it felt like for a Black woman to page through a pregnancy manual and see sections like this: "Will [your baby] have blond hair like Grandma? Green eyes like Grandpa?" Or a skin-care book that describes a rash as turning the skin from pink to red, leaving out the range of shades of Black skin. I pointed to a number of health books targeted to "all women" that showed only photographs and illustrations of white women. "If you're Black and don't see yourself in the pages of a book, it makes you put it down," I said to the editors I met with.

I wrote the book with the National Black Women's Health Project (NBWHP), mentored by the group's founder, the MacArthur genius Byllye Avery. Her organization pointed to a conspiracy of silence in the Black community around both physical and emotional health concerns that made all of our medical problems worse. This silence led to isolation, low self-esteem, and unhealthy lifestyle choices. Byllye, others in the NBWHP leadership, and the activist Angela Y. Davis and the author June Jordan, who wrote the foreword to *Body & Soul,* had been involved in the civil rights and Black Power movements and understood that structural racism and health-care discrimination contributed greatly to the health problems that *Body & Soul* covered. But as a child of the generation that benefited from earlier struggles but was too young to be involved in the movements, I stayed in my sweet spots—information, education, and self-help.

I revised my thinking in the early 1990s when I learned more about the effects of stress on the bodies of mothers and babies during my year at the Harvard School of Public Health, and after having a low-birth-weight baby of my own. I began to think more deeply about the mind-body connection and the link between health and stress. For most of us at that time, stress was synonymous with being stressed-out, which meant having too much to do in too little time. For Black women, this was our burden. In my work at *Essence* and in my books and lectures, I discussed the heavy toll of being "strong" Black women who sacrifice our physical and emotional health to tend to the well-being of others—children, parents, spouses, lovers, elders, friends, the community itself. Around that time, based on a national survey, the California Black Women's Health Project estimated that 60 percent of African American women experienced depression that resulted in weight loss or weight gain, sleep disturbances, lack of energy, feelings of inadequacy, and/or thoughts of suicide or death and escaped through food, smoking, heavy drinking, drug abuse, and unhealthy relationships. Because, the thinking went, it was our responsibility to take care of others, it was our duty to heal ourselves by reducing stress so we could be better caretakers. The best way was through self-love and self-care. Look in the mirror and repeat these words from the (late) poet/playwright Ntozake Shange, I suggested:

i found god in myself
& i loved her
i loved her fiercely.

I also advised exercise, deep breathing, laughing, journaling, exercise, warm baths, and cutting down on or avoiding salt (of course), sugar, red meat, alcohol, caffeine, and refined carbohydrates. "Put down the superwoman cape," I wrote in an article, "and ask for help." None of this advice was wrong and I believe it as strongly today, but this frame is also incomplete.

By the time my daughter was walking, I was starting to come to the realization that the stress that affected the bodies of Black people, particularly Black women, came from more than too much to do in too little time. By then, research had mounted—including early work by Arline Geronimus, ScD, who had coined the term "weathering" to explain the toll of racism on health—pointing to the way stress settles in the body, a bone-deep accumulation of persistent insults and traumatizing life circumstances. Today I'm chagrined to think I believed that the impact of insidious discrimination associated with the lived experience of being Black in America can be washed away in a bubble bath or calmed with journaling or meditation and me time.

To promote my book, I frequently attended events hosted by the National Black Women's Health Project. At a self-help gathering in New York City in the early 1990s, the hundred or so attendees were divided up by race, and the sixty Black women in my group were encouraged to share times when we felt disempowered and unhealthy. I was overwhelmed by what I heard. A woman told the group that she had been rushed to the emergency room, blood gushing from her vagina, because of an IUD embedded in her tissue. When doctors refused to remove it, she yanked it out herself, causing excruciating pain and sterility. Another had a piece of her cervix removed without anesthesia. When she protested, her doctor insisted, "You have no nerve endings down there." One woman wept as she said she had been sterilized without her consent. When I left the room, I felt sad and overwhelmed. I was forced to shift my own philosophy, confronted with the idea that Black people were being harmed and traumatized in health-care settings and that living in America was hurting Black women of all classes and education levels.

Still, I stuck to my empowerment, self-health lens, but now also advising readers of my books and *Essence* to be ferocious as lions when dealing with individual health-care providers who may treat Black patients unfairly. The trick, I believed, was to work within the medical system and squeeze everything you could out of the health-care structure that existed. I rarely challenged that system but advised my audiences to self-advocate for fair treatment. My mantra was "health care is our right and we have to stand up for ourselves and others and get the care we want, deserve, and pay for." I tacked some version of it onto almost everything I wrote—in articles and books—and it was always my coda in lectures about Black health empowerment. I also championed Black physicians and researchers and stressed the importance of having a health-care provider who looked like you. It would take a family medical crisis for me to understand that this advice was insufficient and that our medical system is broken.

In 1999, my father, a college-educated man who had retired from his job as a manager in a division of a federal agency, became critically ill. In his early seventies, he was diagnosed with colon cancer, and as the disease worsened, he also began to suffer from mild dementia. I lived in New York City, across the country from my hometown of Denver, so though my parents had been divorced for years, my mother agreed to manage his care. One day she called me and said, "You need to come home. Your father needs you; he's in the hospital." She instructed me to dress in professional attire and to bring my business cards from *The New York Times,* where I was the editor of the health pages. When she picked me up at the airport, dressed in extremely corporate attire, looking like the hospital vice president she used to be, I asked her, "What are we doing?" Her reply was blunt: "They are treating your father like a n——; we need to let them see who he is."

When we arrived at the veterans' hospital he had insisted on, I was shocked by what I saw: My father—courtly, sophisticated, and always impeccably dressed—was frighteningly thin, disheveled, wearing a dirty hospital gown, his hair uncombed. Worse, he had restraints on his legs. As we walked in, an attendant was speaking to him in a disrespectful hiss. When I pushed past the attendant and leaned down to hug my father, he whispered, "Please get me out of here." Everything changed once we arrived. My mother, flipping into an officious mode I didn't recognize, set everyone straight—doctors, nurses, and hospital administrators. We showed them my father's college degree, medals from his military service, and photographs of him pre-illness. I let his caregivers know that he had studied biology in college, so explaining things in a respectful way would help him understand what was going on and prevent him from feeling afraid and angry. We made them "see" him, beyond his race and the ravages of his illness. My father, who died several months after my mother and I visited him, didn't deserve "special" treatment because of his class and education; class was the only card my mother and I had to play, so we played it. But like anyone, he should've been treated with dignity.

The discrimination and ill-treatment my father suffered as a patient was a deeply personal experience that mirrored the academic understanding I had of health-care bias, and it was a turning point in my work. Over the next two decades of my career in journalism, I would forcefully infuse what I understood about the effects of discrimination on Black health in articles I wrote about HIV/AIDS, diabetes, mental health, and heart disease. In 2017, I got the opportunity to showcase my years of thinking and learning about race, health, and inequality when I spent nearly a year reporting on the crisis in infant and maternal mortality in America. The story followed Simone Landrum, a woman whose medical treatment led to the death of her baby and her own near death. When the story, "The Hidden Toll: Why America's Black Mothers and Babies Are in a Life-or-Death Crisis," was published in April 2018, I was thrilled by the widespread and largely positive response, the feedback, and the actions taken.

After the article ran, book publishers and literary agents approached me about expanding the piece into a book. At first I resisted, and even after I agreed to write this book, I remained quietly unsure that it was necessary. But then something happened to change my mind. In 2018, not long after my article was published, I was invited to a grand rounds with the ob-gyn department of a hospital in a small city in the Midwest. I offered the team of twelve white physicians, who served a large population of women of color, mainly immigrants from East Africa, a snapshot of the article, summarizing the data about racial disparities in infant and maternal mortality.

I explained my theses about the influences of social determinants of health, discrimination in health care, and toxic stress fueled by societal racism. I discussed the circumstances under which Simone Landrum lost her baby daughter and almost lost her life, including having her legitimate concerns dismissed and ignored. I described the callous way nurses and physicians treated her right in front of me as she was delivering her baby son the following year. After I finished, the head of the department was the first to respond. "I don't understand why the medical team let you into the labor and delivery room," he said. "I know I never would've allowed that."

"Wait, that was your takeaway?" I asked him.

For the next half hour, he and his team pushed back against the work I had spent years compiling, unleashing nearly every myth I had painstakingly dispelled in the article, including the idea that genetics were somehow to blame and that Black American women lacked "kinship circles." I was trapped in a game of medical smackdown, dismissing, one by one, their either incorrect or incomplete explanations for the racial disparities in maternal and infant health. Between the lines of their cross-examination, it was clear to me that they were blaming Black American women for the deaths of Black mothers and babies, which they believed could be wiped away with education and more "doctoring," with no regard to the toxic effects of interpersonal and institutional racism. At that moment, in that room of midwestern physicians, I understood that the denial of racial bias can be so extreme that no one believes you even when you have the evidence.

In my years of reporting on public health and race—including interviewing women and men of all classes whose health has been harmed by the medical system and being embedded for months in some of the most disadvantaged communities in the country—not to mention being a slave-descended African American myself, I have seen a race of people who have been mistreated and misunderstood, ignored and blamed, let down and left to fend for ourselves. So we do; we take care of ourselves and each other. This reality shows up in the names and slogans of Black organizations focused on health issues. I wrote about a Black HIV/AIDS services center in D.C. called Us Helping Us, attended a conference called the Saving Ourselves Symposium, and have written about a number of organizations with names like My Brother's Keeper or My Sister's Keeper. These names at once represent empowerment and self-sufficiency but also abandonment. "We are the ones we've been waiting for," long one of the slogans of the Black-led reproductive justice movement, is sometimes paired with a quotation from Fannie Lou Hamer, "I'm sick and tired of being sick and tired."

I remember, a number of years ago, telling my friend Steve Rabin, who is a very smart and thoughtful white man with a long career in health policy and advocacy, about all of the health issues that disproportionately affect African Americans. "That's terrible," he said to me. "How can we solve this problem?" I thought, "We? What does he have to do with it?" "We, Black people, know best how to solve these issues—'our people, our problem, our solution,'" I explained to him, referencing the tagline of the Black AIDS Institute in Los Angeles. "FUBU, for us, by us," I added. "This isn't a FUBU situation or a Black problem," Steve said to me. "This is an American problem, so why should Black people be expected to solve it alone?"

That is what I realized while writing this book: we shouldn't. Since the first African enslaved men, women, and children reached American shores, there has been a Black-white divide in who survives, how they live, and who dies, from birth to the end of life. Despite decades of social, economic, and educational progress and what has unquestionably been the rise of a robust Black middle class, racial health disparities have remained intact. Yes, something about being Black is creating a health crisis, and that something is racism. It is the American problem in need of an American solution.

CHAPTER TWO

THE DANGEROUS MYTH THAT BLACK BODIES ARE DIFFERENT

In the summer of 1973, Minnie Lee Relf and her baby sister, Mary Alice, just fourteen and twelve, were taken from their home in Montgomery, Alabama, cut open, and sterilized against their will and without the consent of their parents by a physician working in a federally funded clinic. The Relf family sought justice, and their case brought shocking awareness to the brutality wrought on the bodies of Black women by medical providers financed by the federal government. The pain the Relf sisters endured also changed the course of history: The lawsuit *Relf v. Weinberger* revealed that 100,000 to 150,000 poor, mostly Black women had been sterilized under U.S. government programs over decades. It also stopped this practice and forced doctors to obtain informed consent before performing sterilization procedures.

What happened to the Relf girls is part of a through line of extreme abuse and disrespect of the Black body at the hands of medical providers in the name of science. It began during slavery and continued after emancipation and into the twentieth century, and remnants of it taint current medical education and practice. J. Marion Sims, MD, who until recently was celebrated as the father of modern gynecology, used Black women as guinea pigs in ways that would be unconscionable today. A slave owner, he practiced painful surgeries without anesthesia on enslaved women in Montgomery, Alabama, between 1845 and 1849. In his autobiography, *The Story of My Life,* Dr. Sims describes the pain the women suffered as he cut their genitals again and again in an attempt to perfect a surgical technique to repair vesicovaginal fistula, which can be a severe complication of childbirth. He described the agony endured by Lucy, one of the women, as "extreme." He performed the operation more than two dozen times on Anarcha, another of the enslaved women. Dr. Sims operated on Lucy, Anarcha, and another woman named Betsey while they knelt, naked, on all fours in front of an audience of doctors, writhing in pain.

Almost a century later, beginning in the early 1930s, scientists recruited Black men to participate in what would become one of the most callous and now infamous episodes in American history, the Tuskegee Syphilis Study. Recruitment flyers read, "Colored People, Do You Have Bad Blood?" In bold print, the advertisements locked in the legitimacy of the "experiment" by offering free blood tests and treatment by the county health department and government doctors. Between 1932 and 1972, the U.S. Public Health Service enrolled 600 men in the study; 399 who had syphilis were part of the experimental group, and 201 were control subjects. Most of the subjects were impoverished sharecroppers who were unable to read. The goal was to examine the progression of untreated syphilis under the assumption that the infection manifested itself differently in Black people—"a notoriously syphilis-soaked race," as physicians and scientists of the time believed. For the Tuskegee Study of Untreated Syphilis in the Negro Male, subjects were told they would receive treatment for their "bad blood," though they never did. In 1943, when penicillin became widely available to treat syphilis, the participants in the study were not offered treatment. Instead, they were poked, prodded, and observed while the illness progressed. Once the men died, doctors autopsied their bodies to compile data on the ravages of the disease.

Late in the era of the syphilis experiment, doctors discovered that rather than bad blood, Henrietta Lacks, a poor Black tobacco farmer and mother of five, had magical cells, so hardy that they were labeled immortal. In 1951, Lacks visited Johns Hopkins Hospital in Baltimore complaining of vaginal bleeding. While she was undergoing treatment for cervical cancer, doctors noticed the resilience of the

cells of her tumor and harvested them without her knowledge or consent. Though she died penniless from the cancer, Lacks's cells—named
HeLa after her—transformed medicine and were bought and sold to
scientists, allowing them to perfect the polio vaccine, gene mapping,
and in vitro fertilization. More than seventy years after her death,
scientists buy HeLa cells and cells with modifications for anywhere
from $400 to thousands of dollars per vial.

In more recent years, our country has faced the sins of the past
and apologized to and sometimes compensated the victims of medical violence. In 1973, Congress held hearings on the Tuskegee Syphilis Study, and the following year the surviving participants and the
heirs of those who died received a $10 million out-of-court settle-
ment. As part of the agreement, the U.S. government promised to
give lifetime medical benefits to living participants, and later wives,
widows, and offspring. Lawmakers stepped up, creating new guidelines to protect human subjects in U.S. government–funded research
projects. In 1997, when issuing a formal apology to the survivors of
the Tuskegee study and the family members of those who died, President Bill Clinton called what the government did "wrong—deeply,
profoundly, morally wrong." Henrietta Lacks also received worldwide recognition. The author Rebecca Skloot brought her story
to light in the 2010 book *The Immortal Life of Henrietta Lacks.* It
became a *New York Times* number one best seller. HBO turned
the book into a movie in 2017, starring Oprah Winfrey as Lacks's
daughter Deborah. In 2018, a statue celebrating Dr. Sims—situated
in Central Park across from the New York Academy of Medicine—
was removed after prolonged protest, including by women wearing
blood-splattered gowns in memory of Anarcha, Betsey, Lucy, and
other enslaved women he abused.

Despite their own history-making sacrifice, the Relf sisters never
got their due. Mary Alice and Minnie Lee live in poverty and obscu-
rity not far from where their fertility was taken from them. Unlike
the survivors of the Tuskegee study and their relatives, the Relfs
never received a presidential apology or a dime. Unlike Lacks, they

didn't get a movie starring Oprah. And unlike J. Marion Sims, the doctors and other health-care providers who were complicit in the sterilization of the Relf girls were not shamed or punished. The two sisters, now in their sixties, live together in a cramped Section 8 apartment behind a strip mall near the Mobile Highway in South Montgomery, scraping by on monthly Social Security checks. They are scarred by what they endured, in their hearts and their bodies. "I can show you what they did to me," Minnie Lee says. She lifts up her T-shirt and reveals a jagged horizontal scar that rips down the center of her belly. "That's where they cut me." As she lowers her shirt—which has the word "courage" printed three times on the front—she drops her head.

Mary Alice, sitting in a chair next to her, watches, her half arm, a disability she was born with, resting lightly on her thigh as she leans in to listen intently to her sister. A speech impediment and intellectual disability make communication difficult for her. "It might have happened a long time ago, but it still brings back memories," Minnie Lee says, looking at her sister. "We're still thinking about it."

In 1972, Jessie Bly, a thirty-year-old Black social worker, was working in downtown Montgomery when she received a call from a local city councilman. Her employer, the City of St. Jude, had been founded by a progressive Catholic priest in the 1930s to serve as a "center for the religious, charitable, educational and industrial advancement of the Negro people." Bly, born and raised in Montgomery, was the daughter of a housekeeper and a grave digger. Her parents understood early that their seventh child was bright and engaged and sent her to private school, and she was the only one of the eight siblings to finish college. Bly returned to Alabama from Europe in the late 1960s with her husband, Ray, an army man who had been transferred to a military base in her home state. Her work at the City of St. Jude included checking on the condition of the elderly and poor to make sure they had necessities and basic services.

That day in 1972, the councilman asked her to take a ride with him to a poor Black community in Montgomery called Flatwood to go see a family. When she asked, "What kind of family?" he replied, "Trust me, in the day that we're living, I never thought that we would see anything like this in the United States of America." In Flatwood, Bly was shocked by what she witnessed. "I was waiting to see a house," she recalls, "but I never saw one." The Relfs, a husband, wife, and three young girls, were living as squatters in a field, sheltered in a shanty built from cardboard boxes. "They had no running water, no electricity," Bly says, closing her eyes and shaking her head as she remembers that first encounter. "I was really taken aback because I just couldn't believe that anybody would be living in those conditions. But they were."

But what Bly says crushed her heart most were the girls, the teenage Katie and her two little sisters, Minnie Lee and Mary Alice. Bly, now a mother, grandmother, great-grandmother, and ordained minister in Montgomery, couldn't shake the image of the youngest girl, who was physically and intellectually disabled. "She was born with an automatic amputation, with the umbilical cord wrapped around her right arm," says Bly. "She had no hand, and the arm was just a little stub."

As she continued meeting with the Relfs, their story began to come together. Like many Black families at the tail end of the Great Migration in the 1950s and 1960s, Lonnie and Minnie Relf, both illiterate, were forced out of rural Macon County in Alabama—ironically, where the Tuskegee Syphilis Study took place. There, cotton was no longer king and mechanization had caused agricultural jobs in the fields to dry up. Like generations before them, some went north, but others crowded into southern cities like Montgomery, the state capital. In 1910, 90 percent of all African Americans lived in the South, three-fourths in rural areas. By 1970, more than half of all Black Americans lived in the North, the vast majority in urban areas. Of those remaining in the South, most now lived in cities. In Alabama specifically, census data shows that for the first time, in 1960, the state's urban population exceeded the size of the rural population in a state that was one-third Black. This influx of rural Blacks, most unskilled and lacking education, increased poverty in Black communities in a number of southern cities like Montgomery.

Bly, desperate to help the Relfs, arranged with the director of the Montgomery Housing Authority for them to live in a three-bedroom apartment in Smiley Court, a public housing project on the southwest side of the city. Once the family moved into their new home, Bly took them to Salvation Army and Goodwill to buy used furniture and put out a call for donations of linens, cooking utensils, and other household items to the people in her church and network. She taught Minnie, who was used to preparing meals on a rudimentary oil burner in old burned pots, how to use a stove and the basics of keeping house. "They didn't know how people really lived," says Bly. "Life had passed them by."

The girls had no idea about hygiene, so Bly showed them how to take care of themselves and got the two older daughters into school. She brought Mary Alice to a pediatrician who specialized in developmental disabilities for evaluation. He declared her mentally incompetent, not teachable but trainable, and recommended the McInnis School for Retarded Children. The diagnostic and guidance clinic he ran was sponsored by the public health service, and now Bly worries that visiting the government-funded facility put the Relf girls on the radar of the family planning clinic that would eventually set up the sterilizations. More likely, they were flagged by the government services they were receiving: food stamps, a $150 monthly welfare check, and a subsidized apartment in public housing. These benefits were lifesaving; even if he'd been able to find a job in Montgomery, Lonnie Relf had been disabled in an accident and was unable to work. The services were administered through the Office of Economic Opportunity (OEO), the federal agency established in 1964 as part of the U.S. government's War on Poverty. Government administrators steered the Relf sisters to the Family Planning Clinic of the Montgomery Community Action Committee, which was also sponsored and controlled by OEO. The U.S. government created its family planning program in 1967 to "help" poor people prevent unwanted births.

The process began with Katie, who was about fifteen when nurses first injected her with Depo-Provera, a contraceptive. At that time, the shots were still in the investigational phase and not yet approved by the FDA for administration to adult women, let alone teenagers. Poor Black women in the South were the overwhelming recipients of the drug under the force of threats of the loss of welfare benefits. The staff at the Family Planning Clinic never obtained permission to perform the injections or adequately explained the shots to Katie or her mother. Some time later, Minnie Lee and Mary Alice also began receiving the shots. A member of the staff would later tell Bly that she was worried that "boys are hanging around the house and we don't want no more of their kind." The implication: they would engage in sexual activity and have children who would require more government benefits, though there was no evidence that any of the girls were sexually active, especially the two younger ones, who hadn't yet reached the teen years. In reality, the Relfs were targeted because of their race and class and because they were judged to be intellectually inferior even though only Mary Alice would be diagnosed with an actual disability. The other two girls simply lacked formal education and were struggling to catch up to their peers. In March 1973, Katie, then seventeen, was again taken to the Family Planning Clinic, this time for insertion of an IUD, after the Food and Drug Administration terminated clinical trials of Depo-Provera because of its link to cancer in animals. Again, though Katie was under the age of consent, her parents say they were not consulted about the IUD.

A few months later, something more sinister happened. On June 13, two nurses came to the Relfs' apartment and informed Minnie that her daughters would need to go to the hospital for what she understood to be more shots. Employed by the Family Planning Clinic, they drove the mother and her two younger daughters first to a doctor's office and then to the Professional Center Hospital in downtown Montgomery. Health-care providers explained that Minnie needed to sign a paper to give consent for treatment. It is unclear what Minnie Relf understood, but she trusted her daughters in the hands of the staff at this clinic, sponsored by the same government that had given her family a home, food, money, and an education for her children. Still, it is very clear that she had no idea that signing the piece of paper would mean that her daughters would never be able to bear children. Since she could not read or write, Minnie signed the surgical consent form with an *X* and was then driven home, while the younger girls remained alone in the ward.

Before Minnie made it home, the same family planning nurse returned to the Relfs' apartment to pick up Katie and bring her to the hospital. The teenager sensed something was wrong and refused to go, locking herself in her room. The following day, Jessie Bly stopped by and a frantic Katie filled her in on what had happened. "Where are your sisters?" Bly asked Katie. "I can show you, Miss Bly," Katie told her, and they got in the car and drove to the Professional Center Hospital.

Even nearly half a century later, Bly has no trouble conjuring the image of the younger Relf girls in the hospital, huddled together, looking small and scared in cotton surgical gowns. The second they saw the social worker, they both began to cry. Clinging to Minnie Lee, a sobbing Mary Alice repeated over and over, "I just hurt so bad. I just hurt so bad, Miss Bly, help me. Help me, Miss Bly."

The violence perpetrated on the Relfs at the hands of health-care providers who should have been helping, not harming, them has its roots in slavery. For centuries, white physicians and scientists went to great lengths to prove that Black people were biologically and physiologically different from white people. They used their expertise and even empirical evidence to create deeply flawed theories, presented as fact, to justify forced labor and unspeakable cruelty and lend support to racist ideology and discriminatory public policies. According to this thinking, Black people were different in mind, body, and even soul, and different meant inferior. The lie that Black men, women, and even children could withstand enormous amounts of pain was the most dangerous, and it provided rationalization for the most vicious aspects of slavery—backbreaking unpaid labor, squalid living conditions, and brutal punishment—in service of keeping the wealth-generating institution alive and thriving. In the 1787 manual *A Treatise on Tropical Diseases: And on the Climate of the West-Indies,* a British doctor, Benjamin Moseley, a member of the Royal College of Physicians in London, claimed that Black people could bear surgical operations much more than white people, noting that "what would be the cause of insupportable pain to a white man, a Negro would almost disregard." To drive home his point in a later edition, he added, "I have amputated the legs of many Negroes who have held the upper part of the limb themselves."

It didn't stop with just physical pain, because, as the false ideas went, Black people didn't feel emotional pain as intensely as whites, justifying separating and selling off enslaved family members. And Black women were raped by their enslavers and other white men, and men and women were forced to reproduce to create a robust supply of free labor under the pseudoscientific notion that Black people were hypersexual, lascivious, and wanton, with genitalia that differed from those of whites, generally perceived as larger.

The genesis of some of this thinking might have been the words of Thomas Jefferson in his influential and widely circulated 1785 book *Notes on the State of Virginia.* Though he was not a doctor or scientist, Jefferson cataloged the physiological ways Black bodies differed from white bodies in this 244-page document. "They have less hair on the face and body," he wrote. "They secrete less by the kidnies [*sic*], and more by the glands of the skin, which gives them a very strong and disagreeable odour. This greater degree of transpiration renders them more tolerant of heat, and less so of cold, than the whites." He also advanced the myth that Black people had weak lungs, justifying hard labor as beneficial. Jefferson, who both owned and fathered enslaved people, extrapolated that Black people were different emotionally and intellectually. "They seem to require less sleep," he wrote. "A black after hard labour through the day, will be induced by the slightest amusements to sit up till midnight, or later, though knowing he must be out with the first dawn of the morning."

"They are more ardent after their female," Jefferson wrote, "but love seems with them to be more an eager desire, than a tender delicate mixture of sentiment and sensation. Their griefs are transient."

Doctors, many who profited from owning enslaved people, grabbed hold of Jefferson's unproven pronouncements and wrapped them in the legitimacy of science. Some southern doctors claimed to be experts in "Negro Medicine," presenting "facts" about Black people not derived from real evidence but pieced together by their own tainted observations. They believed, and went to great lengths to prove, that compared with whites, Blacks had not only higher pain tolerance and weaker lungs but also smaller skulls, better heat tolerance, resistance to some ailments, and susceptibility to others. In his widely read paper "Report on the Diseases and Physical Peculiarities of the Negro Race," Dr. Samuel Cartwright, a New Orleans physician and academic, detailed a laundry list of physical differences between whites and Blacks—including that Blacks had darker blood; harder, whiter bones; smaller brains; and better hearing, smell, and sight than whites. He also suggested that a difference in the nervous systems of Blacks made them, as he put it, value sensuality over intellectuality. "Music is a mere sensual pleasure with the negro," he wrote. "There is nothing in his music addressing the understanding; it has melody, but no harmony; his songs are mere sounds, without sense or meaning—pleasing the ear, without conveying a single idea to the mind; his ear is gratified by sound, as his stomach is by food."

Cartwright took his theories a step further, insisting that slavery benefited Blacks. He believed that a deficiency in cerebral matter and excess of nervous matter distributed to the "organs of sensation and assimilation" created a debasement of the mind, which rendered Blacks childlike, unable to take care of themselves. As a result of these physiological failings, he wrote that slavery gave Black people "more tranquility and sensual enjoyment, [and] expands the mind and improves the morals, by arousing them from that natural indolence so fatal to mental and moral progress."

Cartwright also picked up Jefferson's claim that Blacks have lower lung capacity and saw forced labor as a way to "vitalize the blood" and correct the problem. Enslavement, he argued, offered physiological benefits. "It is the want of a sufficiency of red, vital blood, that chains their mind to ignorance and barbarism, when in freedom," he wrote.

Most outrageously, Cartwright maintained that enslaved people were prone to a disease called drapetomania, which caused them to run away from their masters. Willfully ignoring the inhumane living and working conditions that drove desperate men and women to attempt escape, he insisted, without irony, that enslaved people contracted this ailment when their masters treated them as equals, and he prescribed working them harder or "whipping the devil out of them."

Operating under these erroneous convictions, doctors also routinely bought, sold, and traded enslaved people as research subjects. They were made to suffer excruciating pain in the name of scientific advancement. After death, their bodies—often robbed from graves—were trafficked as cadavers or in pieces for medical students to dissect as part of their training. Under the fallacies of racial physiological differences that southern doctors and scientists were working so hard to advance, John Brown, enslaved on a plantation in Baldwin County, Georgia, during the 1820s and 1830s, was subject to a variety of excruciatingly painful medical experiments and procedures that left him sick and weak, his body disfigured by a network of scars. Brown—or Fed, as his owners called him—had been lent to Dr. Thomas Hamilton, a neighboring physician, who needed a subject to test a cure for sunstroke. After working a full day in the fields, Brown was forced to strip and sit in a pit on a stool resting on a plank just above a hundred-degree fire. Damp blankets were fastened over the hole to make sure heat didn't escape; only his head remained aboveground. As the pit became unbearably hot, Hamilton fed Brown a number of remedies, supposedly to help his body withstand the heat. After about half an hour, Brown would faint and would be lifted out and revived, as the doctor took note of the degree of heat the enslaved man could withstand. Eventually, based on these experiments, Hamilton marketed a remedy for sunstroke. This supposed cure—a pill made from flour combined with a cayenne pepper tea concoction—made him a fortune.

Following the heat experiments, Hamilton became consumed with proving Black-white physiological differences and used Brown to determine how deep Black skin went, believing it was thicker than white skin. Brown, who eventually managed to escape to England, became one of the small number of enslaved people to record his experiences, in an 1855 autobiography, *Slave Life in Georgia: A Narrative of the Life, Sufferings, and Escape of John Brown, a Fugitive Slave, Now in England.* In Brown's own words, Hamilton "appl[ied] blisters to my hands, legs and feet, which bear the scars to this day. He continued until he drew up the dark skin from between the upper and the under one. He used to blister me at intervals of about two weeks." Brown was with Hamilton for a total of nine months until "the Doctor's experiments had so reduced me that I was useless in the field."

Hamilton seems monstrous and his experiments are clearly less scientific than sadistic, but he was actually a courtly southern gentleman, a widely respected physician, and a trustee of the Medical Academy of Georgia. And, like many other doctors of the era in the South, he was also a wealthy plantation owner. Though Cartwright's ideas are preposterous and his 1851 paper reads like satire, he was considered a leader and authority in Negro medicine. Cartwright was a professor of "diseases of the Negro" at the University of Louisiana, which is now Tulane, and served as chair of the committee of Louisiana's medical association that specialized in illness and physiology of the Negro. He presented his theories on Black inferiority, including the drapetomania hypothesis, at the annual meeting of the medical association of Louisiana and his paper was published in

the May 1851 issue of *The New Orleans Medical and Surgical Journal.*
And somehow his theories have managed to stick, and his footprint
remains on modern-day medicine.

Bly was shaken by what had happened to Minnie Lee and Mary
Alice. She recalls being unable to sleep, feeling haunted by the image
of the young girls crying and calling her name as they stood in the
hospital ward. She also worried that this was somehow her fault.
Though she had no clue about the contraceptive shots or the sterilizations, she felt responsible for introducing the girls into the system
in the first place. "I knew I wouldn't be able to rest knowing that this
kind of an injustice had been perpetrated upon these young ladies
and nobody was speaking for them," she says. "It happened because
of where I am, so I felt like God wanted me to be the mouthpiece
for them. I was going to do what I had to do."

After asking around, she was referred to two young civil rights
lawyers, Morris Dees and Joe Levin, who were making their names
as social justice champions. The two attorneys had recently founded
the Southern Poverty Law Center, with the civil rights leader Julian
Bond as its first president, when Jessie Bly walked into their office—
then a small, old house on Washington Avenue in Montgomery that
they had refurbished as a law office. She shared the story of the
Relfs with Levin and Dees, who were outraged but also intrigued.
In July 1973, they filed *Relf v. Weinberger* in federal district court in
Montgomery alleging that "the U.S. Department of Health, Education and Welfare (HEW), now the Department of Health and
Human Services (HHS), was funding the administration of experimental drugs (Depo-Provera) and sterilization procedures under the
guidance of HEW and Office of Economic Opportunity (OEO) to
poor black persons who were dependent upon governmental benefits programs." Caspar Weinberger, the director of HEW from 1973
to 1975, who would later become Ronald Reagan's defense secretary,
was named in the suit. The case was later amended to include two

former White House aides of Richard Nixon's, John W. Dean III and John D. Ehrlichman.

Just before the official filing, Levin picked up the phone and called Julian Bond to brief him on the Relf case. Immediately, Bond saw it as a lightning rod, "a horrendous attack on privacy, innocence and the right of motherhood," he would tell *The New York Times*. He encouraged Levin and Dees to contact the news media. Articles in the *Times* and *Time* magazine and a piece on NBC News shone a white-hot spotlight on the plight of the Relfs and the issue of forced sterilization. "The suit all of a sudden attracted a great deal of attention," remembers Levin. "And it's not that we hadn't had attention but this was actually at a scale that we hadn't seen before."

After she was interviewed by reporters from *The Washington Post* and *Jet* magazine, the media attention became too intense for Bly. "I couldn't go home; I couldn't go to work," she says. "Newspaper, magazine people were following me around to get information, and I had to take my kids and we had to go stay at my mom's for a while."

As publicity about the case increased, Orelia Dixon, the director of the Family Planning Clinic, defended the actions of her facility. In a July 2, 1973, *New York Times* story, Dixon insisted that her nurses were clear when they explained to Minnie Relf that the injections for her daughters were no longer authorized, and suggested sterilization as an alternative. Dixon also explained that she and her staff pushed sterilization as an alternative because the girls were not disciplined enough to take daily birth control pills. "There's no doubt in my mind that they all knew what that meant," Dixon told the *Times*, adding, "We explain everything, and we do not use words that people can't understand." The issue of racism came up when the Relfs' lawyers told the court that the girls had been targeted for sterilization because they were Black. Though Dixon was white, as was the physician who performed the operation, clinic employees noted that the nurses who took the girls from their home were Black.

A *Times* article a few days later included this exchange between Morris Dees and young Minnie Lee:

Q. Are you ever going to get married?
A. Yes.

Q. Are you going to have any children?
A. Yes.

Q. How many?
A. One.

Q. A boy or a girl?
A. A little girl.

The news stories caught the eye of Senator Edward Kennedy, chairman of the Senate Subcommittee on Health of the Committee on Labor and Public Welfare, and he asked Levin and the Relfs to appear before the Senate and tell their story. Bly didn't participate in the hearing, though she knew about it. Her husband had received orders to serve in Germany, and she was preparing to move her family to Frankfurt, where they would live for several years. Levin, along with Lonnie, Minnie, Katie, Minnie Lee, and Mary Alice, flew to Washington—the Relfs' first and only time on an airplane—to testify. Levin and the Relf parents had agreed that it would be too difficult for the girls to speak in an open hearing, so on the morning of July 10, 1973, Katie, Minnie Lee, and Mary Alice met with Kennedy behind closed doors. Levin recalls that the senator showed them pictures of his children, spoke to them gently, and listened closely, moved by what he heard. During the open hearing, Kennedy could barely hide his outrage as he grilled Henry Simmons, MD, HEW's deputy assistant secretary for health and scientific affairs, and other administrators about why the federal government was involved in coercive, nonconsensual sterilizations of Black and poor women. When it was their turn, Lonnie and Minnie stepped tentatively up to the mic to face the senator. Speaking in the gentle tone he had used earlier when meeting with the younger Relfs, Kennedy thanked the parents for appearing and asked them to describe in their own words what had happened to their daughters. They told their story haltingly, Minnie explaining how she had signed an X on the form given to her by the public health service workers. Lonnie insisted, "I didn't want it done, and I'm still upset."

"What was your feeling when you heard that they had operated on your children?" Kennedy asked Mrs. Relf.

"I felt very bad about it," she said. "I got mad."

"Would you have permitted it if you had known about it?" Kennedy asked.

"No," she said. "I would not have let them do that. They said they were going to give the shots."

Kennedy again thanked the Relf family for their testimony, complimenting their three daughters and acknowledging their courage. "We have seen too many mothers and fathers that have been saddened by these kinds of occurrences," Kennedy said. "We are going to do our very best to make sure that it does not happen again."

Levin now says that the Senate testimony and Kennedy's support for the case and issue had an enormous effect. Though the case would take years to resolve, as it made its way through the courts—and the media—a number of things happened. First, the suit helped uncover a pattern of sterilization abuse, financed by the U.S. government and practiced for decades. At the Family Planning Clinic that executed the sterilizations of the Relf children, eleven other teenage girls had been sterilized, ten of them Black. But the practice turned out to be even more widespread. In July 1973, the same month Levin and Dees first filed the Relfs' case, a Black woman from North Carolina, Nial Ruth Cox, also filed a suit against a doctor who had surgically sterilized her after telling her that the results would "wear off." At the time of the sterilization in 1965, Cox was eighteen, unmarried, and the mother of a baby girl. Cox lived with her mother, who was a recipient of government benefits. A governmental caseworker threatened to strike the family from the welfare rolls unless the mother agreed to have her daughter's tubes tied temporarily. Five years later, Cox would learn that the sterilization was permanent. Though Cox—who was represented by several lawyers,

including the future Supreme Court justice Ruth Bader Ginsburg—
lost in court, her suit revealed that her sterilization was part of a
eugenics program that had begun decades before. In North Carolina, doctors performed some 7,600 sterilizations between 1933 and
1974, justified as a way to keep welfare rolls low, reduce poverty,
and improve the gene pool by preventing the "mental deficient"
from reproducing. The vast majority of those sterilized in that state
were Black. Like North Carolina, thirty-one other states had eugenics programs. Government-sanctioned sterilization has extended
beyond Black women and includes women of other races. In California, more than 17,000 women of Mexican descent were sterilized
between 1920 and 1945 under a U.S. eugenics law used to prevent
reproduction of those deemed "unfit." In 1976, a study by the U.S.
General Accounting Office found that between 1973 and 1976, four
of the twelve Indian Health Service regions sterilized 3,406 Native
American women without their permission, including three dozen
who were under twenty-one. The same year, HEW reported that
over 37 percent of Puerto Rican women of childbearing age, most
in their twenties, had been sterilized between the 1930s and the
1970s. The U.S. government had been involved in population control beginning in 1898, when it assumed governance of Puerto Rico,
worried that overpopulation would increase poverty and other social
and economic conditions.

Eventually, because of the Relfs' case and others, the hearings and
the media unearthed an estimated 100,000 to 150,000 poor, mostly
Black women sterilized each year in the United States under federally
funded programs. Many others were coerced into sterilization when
health-care providers threatened to cut off their benefits unless they
agreed to give up their fertility. The Relfs' suit ended these practices,
and HEW was forced to withdraw regulations under which the government funded forced sterilizations. The federal government also
created a requirement that health-care providers obtain informed
consent—more than the X Minnie Relf signed—before performing
sterilization procedures.

Before the case came to a close in 1977, Levin and Dees wanted to help out the Relf family, who were still living on the margins in the same public housing apartment, subsisting on monthly checks from the government. Neither attorney had much experience in personal injury law, so they recruited Melvin Belli to file a damages suit to compensate the Relfs. Belli, nicknamed King of Torts—and Melvin Bellicose by insurance companies—was an unlikely choice to handle the Relf case. Loud, outrageous, and flamboyant, Belli was best known for his celebrity clients: Errol Flynn, Mae West, Lana Turner, Lenny Bruce, Zsa Zsa Gabor, Muhammad Ali, and the Rolling Stones. In 1964, Belli first reached celebrity status himself by defending Jack Ruby after Ruby shot Lee Harvey Oswald, John F. Kennedy's assassin. Belli's firm filed a $5 million damages suit on behalf of the Relfs in February 1974 and, after it was dismissed, upped the ante with another suit for $15 million in July of that same year. This suit would have obviously offered a tectonic reversal of fortunes for the Relf family.

Accounts of medical violence dating back to slavery and outlandish, supposedly scientific theories by physicians like Cartwright are greeted with shock and presented as a throwback to the past or as an aberration, the work of a few bad actors. Still, the concept of biological and psychological differences based on race and some of the deeply questionable medical theories and practices from slave times have clung stubbornly to the present, normalized in today's medical theory and practice. Even today the centuries-old fallacies of Black immunity to pain and weakened lung function still show up. At the same time, scientists and doctors ignore or downplay the social and environmental conditions that mar Black lives and communities, and overlook the dark history of racial prejudice based on the assumption of inherent Black inferiority that has poisoned the U.S. health-care system. Even Cartwright's fabrications somehow remain embedded in current medical practice. To validate his theory about lung deficiency in African Americans, he became one of the first American doctors to measure pulmonary function with an instrument called a spirometer. Using a device he designed himself, Cartwright estimated that "the deficiency of the Negro may be safely estimated to be 20 percent." Today, most commercially available spirometers, used by medical providers around the world to diagnose and monitor respiratory illness, have a "race correction" built into the software, which controls for the false notion that Black people have less lung capacity than whites. In her book *Breathing Race into the Machine: The Surprising Career of the Spirometer from Plantation to Genetics,* the Brown University professor Lundy Braun notes that race correction is standard practice, treated as fact in textbooks and still taught in many medical schools.

For a variety of illnesses, surgeries, and other medical procedures, in the emergency room and during childbirth, numerous studies have found that Black people receive less evaluation for pain and less relief from it compared with people of other races. Recent data shows that present-day doctors neglect to sufficiently treat the pain of Black adults and children for a variety of medical issues. A 2013 review of studies examining racial disparities in pain management published in the American Medical Association's *Virtual Mentor* found that Black and Hispanic people—from children receiving tonsillectomies to elders in hospice care—received inadequate pain management compared with their white counterparts. The research noted that in some cases the more severe the pain, the wider the disparity in treatment. As recently as 2016, a survey of 222 white medical students and residents published in *The Proceedings of the National Academy of Sciences* showed that half of them endorsed at least one myth about physiological differences between Black people and white people, including that Black people's nerve endings are less sensitive than whites'. When asked to imagine how much pain white or Black people experienced in situations like getting their hands slammed in a car door, the medical students and residents insisted that Black people felt less pain, which made the providers less likely to recommend appropriate treatment. About 40 percent of first- and second-year medical students and 25 percent of residents believed the lie that Thomas Hamilton tortured John Brown to prove: that Black skin is thicker than white skin.

This disconnect between what is known and what many scientists, doctors, and other medical providers—and those training to fill their positions in the future—still believe allows them to ignore their own complicity in health-care inequality. Their insistence on belief in racial difference as science lets them dismiss internalized racism and both conscious and unconscious bias as forces that drive them to go against their oath to do no harm.

The Relf case happened almost fifty years ago, in another century, and many insist that it was a dark moment in history that could never happen now. But coerced contraception, including sterilization, at the hands of physicians and other health-care providers has continued in various forms. In 2013, the Center for Investigative Reporting found that physicians under contract with the California Department of Corrections and Rehabilitation sterilized nearly 150 female inmates from 2006 to 2010 without required state approvals. At least 148 women received tubal ligations in violation of prison rules during those five years. State documents and interviews pointed to some 100 more dating back to the late 1990s. From 1997 to 2010, the state paid doctors $147,460 to perform the procedure, according to a database of contracted medical services for state prisoners. In 2017, Judge Sam Benningfield of White County, Tennessee, was reprimanded for promising thirty-day sentence reductions to incarcerated men and women who agreed to receive vasectomies or birth control implants. Benningfield claimed he was trying to encourage personal responsibility and prevent incarcerated people from being burdened with children when they were released. Civil rights attorneys called the program both "an unconstitutional, coercive intrusion on the rights of vulnerable people and a modern-day eugenics scheme." It hasn't ended: In the fall of 2020, a nurse at a for-profit Immigration and Customs Enforcement detention center in Georgia reported that unnecessary gynecological procedures—including hysterectomies—had been performed on immigrant women. The women said that they had undergone the surgeries without fully understanding or consenting to them.

Even after the Relf case created changes in laws, regulations, and guidelines regarding forced or coerced sterilization, the damages suit ushered through the courts by Melvin Belli dragged on, mired in mountains of paperwork and technicalities—motions, reversals, reconsiderations, and transfers. The Relfs' damages suit finally ended, dismissed on a technicality in January 1977 with the family, still penniless, receiving no money. "I felt sorry for them, the kids and family," Joe Levin says now. "The issue was brought to light but had no beneficial consequences for the kids and the Relf family. It felt very bad."

Two states that were part of the government's long-running eugenics plot stepped up and compensated their victims. In 2013, North Carolina, where Nial Ruth Cox's suit shined a harsh light on that state's eugenics program, agreed to give victims of forced or coerced sterilization financial compensation, setting aside up to $50,000 per individual. Virginia followed in 2015 and gave each surviving victim $25,000. Though California apologized to the victims of its eugenics program in 2003, none of the other states have acknowledged the pattern of sterilization of poor and mostly Black women, and the federal government has remained silent regarding its role in providing funding.

The Relfs have been left out in the cold. Minnie Lee never finished high school, dropping out in the eleventh grade. Keeping up with classwork was difficult for her, given the absence of formal learning in her early childhood and the limitations of her parents. "I was a slow reader in school," she says now. "I can read, but I'm just slow. I was just slow."

She also recalls her classmates making fun of her. "People was just picking at me at school, always saying, 'You can't have no children. You can't do this and you can't . . .'" she says, her voice trailing off. "It hurt me. I felt so sad."

Mary Alice did end up in McInnis, the special needs school that Jessie Bly had sought out for her. But she didn't graduate either. Both women remember that Mary Alice spent several years in foster care, living with a woman named Ms. Dot. Their mother died in 1980, just as they reached womanhood, and their father passed away in 2009. Katie, their older sister, lives nearby in another home in the same complex, and they also have other family, including several other siblings. But it's mostly the two of them, walking to the store together for groceries, attending church, sitting side by side watching TV—bound together by love, blood, hurt, and trauma. "Some days I feel sad, but other times just tired," says Minnie Lee, who explains that she and her sister struggle with hypertension and asthma. Mary Alice also suffers from seizures. "Not long ago, I was crying and felt like doing something to myself, like I wanted to go with my mom and dad," Minnie Lee adds, looking over at her sister, who doesn't seem to understand.

They survived the injustice but cannot grasp the importance of their sacrifice or the way it changed history. Minnie Lee recalls the lawsuit; Dees, Levin, and of course Miss Jessie; the trip to D.C. and Senator Kennedy. But when I describe the impact of their case, Minnie Lee looks confused, her face slack. Mary Alice holds on to my arm and smiles. Minnie Lee may not understand what the world gained because of the Relf case, but she is crystal clear about what she and Mary Alice lost. Each woman sleeps with a brown baby doll, Mary Alice's nestled in a tangle of sheets, Minnie Lee's laid across her pillow. These are the shadows of the children that were stolen from them. "I know I can't have kids, and it gets to me sometimes," explains Minnie Lee. "Every time I see somebody like my cousin or my niece Debbie with their child, I think about it. Seeing these little pretty babies, I wish that was me."

CHAPTER THREE

UNEQUAL TREATMENT

The Relf case happened in another century, but reports of racial bias in health care remain distressingly common. Though they are often dismissed as an aberration or the work of a few bad players, in fact piles of data, including research published in the world's top science journals, exhaustive reports by government agencies and non-profit organizations, and evidence revealed during legal actions, all point to a medical system riddled with deeply rooted bias and discrimination, most of it implicit, that affects people the second they venture into our health-care system. Though the problem has been well documented, each new report is met with shock and surprise. After an initial media splash and a round of outrage, the evidence recedes into history, failing to drive significant action or policy. That leaves questions of discrimination in the health-care system ignored, denied, under-examined, misunderstood, and tragic.

Because of the way I saw my father treated by health-care providers in 1999, this issue is far from academic for me, and I understand from my personal vantage the real-world consequences. Nearly twenty years later, in the process of reporting a 2018 *New York Times Magazine* cover story, "Why America's Black Mothers and Babies Are in a Life-or-Death Crisis," I would witness another instance of mistreatment of a Black person by medical providers who were tasked with a bare minimum of "first, do no harm."

The story came to me by happenstance. One Saturday afternoon in the late spring of 2017 during my weekly pickup soccer game in

Brooklyn, Katrina Anderson, who was then a lawyer with the Center for Reproductive Rights in New York City—and a very good soccer player—suggested I write an article about women who die or almost die related to pregnancy and childbirth. Her organization had recently collaborated with the reproductive justice group Sister-Song in Atlanta to form the Black Mamas Matter Alliance, which was tasked with bringing attention to what she referred to as the growing crisis of maternal mortality. As she pitched me her idea for a feature in the *Times* magazine, where I had just become a contributing writer, I argued her down, using all of the familiar assumptions about racial health disparities. "Maternal mortality is a problem of poor countries, a concern of another era," I said, attempting to pry myself loose from her to enjoy the sunny day and fresh air. "American women hardly ever die in childbirth anymore."

"No, I'm talking about today, in our country," she insisted.

"Well, in the U.S., only extremely poor women die related to pregnancy and childbirth," I argued.

But she grabbed my arm and insisted, "Actually, the United States is the only wealthy country where the numbers of women who die or almost die related to pregnancy and childbirth are increasing. This problem is driven by the deaths of Black women. Didn't you used to work at *Essence* magazine?" She refused to allow me to look away as she continued. "Did you know that a Black woman with an advanced degree is more likely to die related to pregnancy and childbirth, or almost die, than a white woman with an eighth-grade education? Don't you have a master's degree?" She had my attention. Several weeks later, the *Times* magazine assigned me the story.

Over the next few months, I set out to understand why in our country with the most expensive and advanced medical technology in the world, growing numbers of American women, disproportionately Black women, were dying as a result of pregnancy and childbirth, including African American women whose income and education should protect them. I collected reams of studies and interviewed at least thirty medical experts, historians, and advocates. To keep the story more hopeful and inspirational and less frightening and depressing, I decided to lift up the work of doulas, people, generally women, who are trained to advocate and support women during pregnancy, labor, delivery, and in the weeks after the birth of a baby. As with other health-care providers grouped under the catchall term "community health workers," I saw their work as one solution to the crisis and began looking for an individual or group who worked with women of color and accepted clients regardless of their ability to pay to use as a narrative thread to wrap around the data, studies, and interviews I had gathered. At the Decolonizing Birth Conference in Brooklyn in September 2017, a convening of health-care providers, researchers, and activists interested in reproductive and birth justice, I got lucky. One of my sources tracked me down at the meeting of about two hundred people and pointed to a striking young Black woman wearing a T-shirt with an abstract swirl of a pregnant belly on the front. She was surrounded by a mixed-race group of women wearing the same shirt and juggling several babies and toddlers. "That's Latona Giwa," my source explained. "She's trained as a labor and delivery nurse but became disenchanted with the medical system and started a social justice doula collective in New Orleans." By the end of the day, Latona had invited me to New Orleans to learn more about her work with the Birthmark Doula Collective and shadow her for a week.

Because I was working full-time as a college professor, it took me several months to synthesize my reporting and pull together a rough draft of my article. So, by the time I was ready to join Giwa in New Orleans, other media outlets had begun to cover the issue, largely thanks to the advocacy of the Black Mamas Matter Alliance. What I noticed in most of the other pieces, however, was a disconnect between the uptick in the deaths of American women in childbirth—including the disproportionate number of Black women who were dying or almost dying—and the racial gap in infant mortality. One widely read, celebrated, and well-executed investigation on maternal mortality that rolled out while I was still deep in the reporting on my article focused on a white nurse who had tragically died in childbirth. This piece, part of Lost Mothers, an excellent multimedia series produced by journalists from ProPublica and NPR, seemed to blame her death—and the maternal mortality crisis—on a hyper focus on saving babies using advancements in neonatal technology, at the expense of their mothers. Though it made sense on the surface, that framework assumed that maternal mortality was largely a clinical/technical problem that could be remedied with clinical/technical solutions. But given my knowledge about the ongoing crisis of low-birth-weight, preterm births and infant mortality among Black babies—and my own low-birth-weight baby girl despite my good health and gold-standard health care—the idea that Black mothers were on the losing end of a tug-of-war with their babies in the delivery room didn't make sense to me. According to that theory, as more Black mothers were dying, shouldn't more and more Black babies be saved? In fact, as I was reporting, I came across a paper in the journal *JAMA Pediatrics* that noted that despite sustained progress in reducing the overall infant mortality rate in America over the previous two decades, in 2014 the Black rate had started to inch up even as the white rate continued its decline. What's more, my friend Dána-Ain Davis, an anthropologist and doula who has written extensively about reproductive justice, pointed me to statistics that showed the racial disparity in infant mortality was actually greater in the present day than in 1850, when Black women were human chattel and babies of all races died so frequently that parents hesitated to name them.

As I tried to think through my story, a quotation from Fannie Lou Hamer came to mind: "A Black woman's body was never hers alone." I began to ask doctors and researchers a different set of questions—not just about maternal mortality, but about the connection between the deaths of mothers and the deaths of their babies. I knew that prenatal care alone had not been enough to spare my daughter from being born smaller than expected. Could something be going on with Black women's bodies that began even before pregnancy that affected not just the mother's health but also the health of her baby? I also thought hard about the racial disparities in the deaths and near deaths of both mothers and infants: Why were Black women three to four times more likely to die and Black infants twice as likely to die compared with white mothers and infants? Why is the current Black-white disparity in both maternal and infant mortality widest at the upper levels of education? And what was it about our health-care system that exacerbated this problem?

As my reporting continued, I realized that the interwoven crises of Black maternal and infant mortality offered me a chance to explore decades of data about the connection between societal racial discrimination, bias in our health-care system, and racial health disparities. I slogged my way through dozens of studies and the footnotes of those studies examining the ways toxic stress, triggered by discrimination, affected the bodies of Black women, which I will discuss in the next chapter of this book. I also assembled a large and damning file of studies and reports about racial bias and mistreatment of Black patients in the health-care system dating back to slavery. I was homing in on a new understanding of what was going on in maternal and infant mortality, laying out how discrimination and bias led to a disproportionate number of poor birth outcomes in Black women. The well-being of American mothers and babies matters: it determines the health of the next generation and can predict future public health challenges for families and communities.

I was particularly intrigued by studies out of Columbia University. Over the years, international researchers have gathered copious examples of disrespect and abuse of women during childbirth, primarily in developing countries. These include shouting at, scolding, or humiliating patients; requesting bribes; conducting medical procedures without consent; and detaining mothers and babies for the inability to pay. Women have also reported being slapped, pinched, hit, or tied down while in labor. Needless to say, this kind of mistreatment erodes trust and drives pregnant women in poor countries away from delivering their babies in health-care facilities.

Lynn Freedman, director of the Averting Maternal Death and Disability Program at Columbia University's Mailman School of Public Health, decided to apply the lessons she and her colleagues learned studying disrespect and abuse in maternal care in

Tanzania—where problems in pregnancy and childbirth lead to nearly 20 percent of deaths occurring in women aged fifteen to forty-nine—to her own backyard, New York City. Freedman, a Harvard-trained former practicing attorney, explained to me that disrespect and abuse mean more than just somebody not being nice to another individual person. "There is something structural and much deeper going on in the health system that then expresses itself in poor outcomes and sometimes deaths."

Though the study had not been completed in 2017 when I was reporting my story, early focus groups made up of some fifty women who recently delivered babies in Washington Heights and Inwood, and of doulas who work in both Washington Heights and central Brooklyn, revealed a range of grievances—from being ignored, scolded, and demeaned to feeling bullied or pushed into having C-sections. For example, most women in the study had to wait one to two months before an initial prenatal appointment, not because they didn't understand the importance of proper care during pregnancy, but due to a lack of availability. After she finally received an appointment, one pregnant woman says she sat in a clinic waiting area from 10:00 a.m. to almost 6:00 p.m.

In another instance, when a laboring woman cried out in pain, a nurse told her, "No one is forcing you to have children [so] you shouldn't be complaining." Another, also in the throes of labor, was asked, "Why do you have so many kids anyway? Mexican women do nothing but have kids here." A doula reported that when her client squatted to alleviate pain during labor—a suggested practice all over the world—a health-care provider said, "We don't do that here; do you think we're in the jungle of Africa?"

In November 2017, I made it to New Orleans to shadow Latona Giwa. On a sunny Friday, the air thick with humidity, she and I pulled up to the home of her twenty-three-year-old client, Simone Landrum. Landrum lived in Broadmoor, a section of New Orleans that battled back from a green dot designation, which meant the community was initially destined to be abandoned after Katrina, razed instead of rebuilt. Still dealing with the aftershocks of a traumatic delivery the previous year that ended in the death of her baby daughter, Harmony, and nearly took her life, Landrum was thirty-two weeks pregnant, fragile, and afraid. She had connected with Giwa, who worked with her pro bono, through a nonprofit organization that provided services for survivors of domestic violence and sexual assault. Landrum sought the group's help after fleeing an abusive relationship. Once counselors explained the role of a doula, Landrum, who also had two young sons, requested one; her primary goal was to avoid going through pregnancy and childbirth alone.

Giwa walked up the steps and reached toward the doorbell, then thought twice about the shrill sound and called her client instead. Landrum opened the door, relieved to see the smiling, fresh-scrubbed Giwa, a lissome slip of a woman, who at thirty-one looked years younger than her client. I followed Landrum and Giwa through the living room, empty save a tangle of disconnected cable cords lying on the bare floor like black snakes. She left behind most of her belongings when she managed to get away from her abusive partner. The two women sat at the kitchen table, where Giwa reviewed her client's last doctor visit, prodding her for details—her blood pressure and weight as well as the baby's size and position.

Landrum shared the story of her stillborn baby and her own brush with death with Giwa and me in fits and starts. In the spring of 2016, she remembers feeling tired and both nauseated and ravenous at the same time and knew she was pregnant. But as her pregnancy progressed, she noticed something different this time. The trouble began with constant headaches and sensitivity to light. Landrum described the pain as "shocking." As her January due date grew closer, she noticed that her hands and feet were swollen and her face looked "puffy" in selfies that she posted on Instagram. But her doctor brushed aside her complaints, recommending Tylenol for the headaches. At a prenatal appointment on November 11, 2016, a few days before her baby shower, Landrum told her doctor that the headache had intensified and Tylenol did not help and that she also felt achy and tired. A handwritten note from the appointment, sandwiched into a printed file of her electronic medical records that she and I would later track down, shows an elevated blood-pressure reading of 143/86. Combined with headaches, swelling, and fatigue, the reading should've pointed to the possibility of preeclampsia, dangerously high blood pressure during pregnancy. High blood pressure and cardiovascular disease are two of the leading causes of maternal death, and hypertensive disorders during pregnancy had been on the rise over the previous two decades. Preeclampsia and eclampsia, the seizures that develop after preeclampsia, are more common in Black women than women of other races.

At the appointment, when Landrum complained more forcefully about how she was feeling, her doctor told her to lie down and scolded her to "calm down." He also warned her that he was planning to go out of town and told her that if she wished, he could deliver the baby by C-section that day, six weeks before her early January due date. Landrum says it felt like an ultimatum, centered on his schedule and convenience. Aside from the handwritten note, Landrum's medical records don't mention the hypertensive episode, the headaches, or the swelling, and she says that was the last time the doctor or anyone from his office spoke to her. Later she would tell me that she felt as though "he threw me away."

Four days later, Landrum had a severe backache and felt so tired she couldn't get out of bed. That evening, she packed a bag and asked her boyfriend to take her sons to her stepfather's house and then drive her to the hospital. In the car on the way to drop off the boys, she felt wetness between her legs and assumed her water had broken. But when she looked at the seat, she saw blood. By the time she was lying on a gurney in the emergency room of Touro, the public hospital located in uptown New Orleans, the splash of blood had turned into a steady stream. In the ER, with doctors and nurses hovering over her, everything became both hazy and chaotic. Her medical records show that her blood pressure had shot up to 160/100. When a nurse moved a monitor across her belly, Landrum couldn't hear a heartbeat. She remembers asking the nurse, "Is she okay? Is she all right?" but nobody said a word. The emergency room doctor dropped his head and then looked into her eyes and explained that the baby was dead inside her. Landrum then turned her head to the side and threw up.

Sedated but conscious, Landrum felt her mind growing foggy. She felt exhausted, like giving up. But then she pictured the faces of her two young sons and thought, "Who's going to take care of them if I'm gone?" That's the last thing she recalls clearly. When she became more alert some time later, a nurse told her that she had almost bled to death and had required half a dozen units of transfused blood and platelets to survive. A few hours later, a nurse brought Harmony, who had been delivered stillborn via C-section, to her. Wrapped in a hospital blanket, her hair thick and black, the baby looked peaceful, as if she were dozing. Landrum recalls holding her, and through the sedation wondered, "Why doesn't she wake up?" Later, she felt angry and thought, "Why is God doing this to me?"

The hardest part was going to pick up her sons empty-handed and telling them that their sister had died. Choking up, she explained to me that she felt as if something had been taken from her, but also from them.

As we sat across the table from each other, I was extremely moved by Landrum's story and grateful that she had had the wherewithal to tell me, in graphic detail, what had happened to her. For me, she offered a real-life example of what happens when the twin and inter-related crises of infant and maternal mortality land in the body of one woman. I felt a rush of empathy for her when later in the visit she expressed strong and legitimate fears about what might happen during the birth of the baby inside her, given her traumatic experience from only a year ago. Though she was scheduled to deliver this baby at a different hospital and with a new ob-gyn, a woman this time, she was still terrified. "I'm trying not to be worried, but sometimes . . ." she said haltingly, looking down at the table. "I feel like my heart is so anxious."

Giwa, with her calming tone and sensitive physical touch, worked to talk through and ease her client's anxiety. As Landrum let loose a litany of her fears—rumors about the hospital where she heard "they kill people," bleeding again during labor, coming home empty-

handed, worries about dying and leaving her sons motherless—
Giwa leaned across the table, speaking evenly with a kind of sis-
terly spirituality. "I know that it was a tragedy, and a huge loss
with Harmony," she said, "but don't forget that you survived, you
made it, you came home to your sons." Giwa then handed Landrum a crayon from the bag she had brought with her, purple,
Landrum's favorite color. She suggested they write affirmations for
Landrum to post, one on the fridge, another on the bathroom mirror. As Landrum scribbled some of her worries in tight, tiny letters,
Giwa wrote down an affirmation for her to post. "I know God has
his arms wrapped around me and my son," Giwa wrote in large
purple letters, outlining "God" and "arms" in red, as Landrum
watched. She took out another sheet of paper and wrote, "Harmony
is here with us, protecting us." After the period, she drew two purple
butterflies. Landrum's eyes locked on the butterflies. "Every day, I
see a butterfly, and I think that's her. I really do," she said. For the
first time, I saw Landrum's shoulders drop.

As I was leaving after our two-hour visit, I thanked Landrum
and hugged her, feeling a real connection, grateful for her honesty,
inspired by her courage, and angered by the callous treatment that
most likely resulted in Harmony's death and Landrum's near death.
As I untangled myself from the embrace, I noticed Landrum looking at me intently. Something told me to ask, "Who will be with
you when you have the baby this time?" "Just me and the doula," she
said. Impulsively, I told her, "I'll be there too," and she smiled. I had
had two children of my own, and had attended the births of my two
godchildren, so it might be nice for her to have another supportive
person by her side during labor. I also figured I would write a first
draft of my story, then return to New Orleans to be with her during her delivery and add what I hoped would be a happy ending to
the piece. I had no idea that what would happen to Landrum in the
delivery room—and the treatment I would observe—would actually
turn out to be the heart-gripping centerpiece of my article.

—

Many thought the attention paid to a 1999 study published in *The New England Journal of Medicine* would cause doctors and other health-care providers to face up to their own bias at work. Rarely has an article with a title as dry as "The Effect of Race and Sex on Physicians' Recommendations for Cardiac Catheterization" received as much notice and generated as much controversy. The study, published in the February 25, 1999, issue of the journal, addressed the issue of physician bias directly and was the first large-scale study to do so focusing exclusively on treatment decisions made by doctors.

Kevin A. Schulman, MD, a physician with an MBA from Wharton and an interest in health services research and policy, and his colleagues chose this topic for a reason: Blacks in the United States have the highest rate of hypertension, with more than half affected, and African Americans aged eighteen to forty-nine are twice as likely as whites to die from heart disease. But studies had shown they are less likely than other groups to be referred for cardiac catherization when complaining of chest pain. Cardiac "cath" is a common procedure used to evaluate heart function in order for heart specialists to diagnose coronary artery disease and to decide whether to perform cardiac surgery.

To understand the role of race in this decision making, Dr. Schulman developed a standardized computer program that included videotaped interviews with patients—two Black men, two Black women, two white men, and two white women—but unbeknownst to the physicians taking part in the study, the patients were actually eight actors, dressed in the same generic hospital gown, reading from identical scripts. The researchers standardized most aspects of the patients' medical and social histories; half were fifty-five, half seventy years old. All had the same insurance and the same occupation—assembly supervisor for the fifty-five-year-old patients, retired assembly supervisor for the seventy-year-olds. Each patient had a father who had had a heart attack at age seventy-five. The 720 participating physicians, the majority of them white men, took part in the survey at two different national medical conferences.

The researchers found that men and whites had a significantly higher probability of being referred for cardiac catheterization than women and Blacks. The largest gap was between Black women and white men, who served as the reference category. The study never accused doctors, nurses, and other health-care providers of being racist. Instead, they concluded that while multiple factors influence physicians' decisions, bias and stereotypes cannot help but play a role. "Bias may represent overt prejudice on the part of physicians," they wrote, "or, more likely, could be the result of subconscious perceptions rather than deliberate actions or thoughts. Subconscious bias occurs when a patient's membership in a target group automatically activates a cultural stereotype in the physician's memory regardless of the level of prejudice the physician has."

The minute the findings became public, Dr. Schulman, who was still early in his career, found himself in the glare of the media spotlight and at the center of feverish controversy. Though the role of what is now generally called implicit bias in medical care is widely acknowledged as a problem today, twenty years ago it was barely recognized in the fields of medicine and science, which were assumed to be purely objective and color-blind. ABC's *World News This Morning* warned viewers, "How your doctor treats your heart may depend on the color of your skin." *Nightline* devoted an entire segment to the study, introducing it this way: "Last night we told you how the town of Jasper, Texas, is coming to terms" with the racially motivated murder of a Black man. "Tonight we will focus on [doctors] who would be shocked to learn that what they do routinely fits quite easily into the category of racist behavior." Aubrey Lewis, MD, a Black cardiologist who appeared on the segment, noted that "if this continues on, you're looking at literally a decimation of the African American population." An editorial in the British medical journal *The Lancet* characterized the results "as close to a definition of institutionalized racism as doctors and health care providers may dare to get."

The backlash was nearly as swift. Physicians and scientists took offense, criticizing Dr. Schulman and his associates over their statistical methods, reporting of the results, and interpretation of the findings. Five months after publication of the study, a group of doctors from Dartmouth Medical School accused Dr. Schulman of exaggerating the findings, which, they wrote in the July 22, 1999, issue of *The New England Journal of Medicine,* "serves to fuel anger and undermine the trust between physicians and their patients." The journal editors also published a note in the same issue, taking responsibility for the media's "over-interpretation of the original article"—though they had vetted the statistical measure before publishing the work. Even as the controversy swirled and the scientists bickered about statistics, in October of that year a survey published by the Henry J. Kaiser Family Foundation found that African Americans were more than twice as likely as whites to state that discrimination in health care is a major problem, almost three times as likely to report that African Americans receive lower-quality health care, and fourteen times as likely to report that they had been treated unfairly because of race when seeking medical care in the recent past.

I spoke to Dr. Schulman, now a professor of medicine at the Stanford University School of Medicine, in 2020 about the 1999 study, and he continues to be proud of his work, unmoved by the criticism. He recalls President Bill Clinton being intrigued and inspired by the study, which he encouraged his cabinet members to read. In 2000, Clinton signed legislation establishing the National Center on Minority Health and Health Disparities to take a deeper dive into the issues Dr. Schulman had unearthed. Dr. Schulman also provided congressional testimony about physician bias along with the African American doctors Louis Sullivan, MD, and David Satcher, MD. Dr. Schulman says he remains most moved by an experience shared by Bennie Thompson, a congressman from Mississippi who came of age in the 1950s, during a closed-door session with the Congressional Black Caucus in 2000. "When he was growing up in Mississippi, no white doctor would ever touch a Black patient," Dr. Schulman recalled. "So, my work wasn't surprising to him or any of them in the room."

—

As Landrum's December 21, 2017, due date moved closer, I stayed in touch with Giwa from New York City, where I live. Landrum was doing fine, but Giwa expected her to go into labor early, since that's what had happened with her other pregnancies. I kept a bag packed so I could jump on a plane and get to New Orleans once her labor started. On Saturday, December 9, Giwa texted me that she thought Landrum was in early labor. I was reading the text at a very raucous holiday party and managed to sober up and call Giwa. "I think you should get here in the next forty-eight hours," she told me. I somehow pulled it together and got a ticket to fly to New Orleans early the next morning. As I was boarding the flight, I received a text from Giwa: "May be a false alarm. Cramping and discomfort have died down for now."

I went anyway. I rented an Airbnb a few blocks from Landrum and spent the next week and a half driving her to doctor's appointments, taking her for walks, and cooking dinner for her and the kids as we waited for the baby to come. "This is not what I expected, but I'm going with it," I told Giwa. During that time, Landrum and I got to know each other better, and we discovered that we had a similar sense of humor and no sense of direction and the same taste in mushy rom-coms. I was also able to share some of my reporting on maternal and infant mortality and the connection to race and discrimination with her. She was very inquisitive and interested in the experts I had interviewed who were studying the issue. "White people care about this, for real?" she asked me.

A few days before her due date, I took Landrum to the hospital for her last ultrasound before the birth. Because of the stillbirth the previous year, her doctor did not want to let the pregnancy go past forty weeks, to avoid the complications that can come with post-term delivery, so an induction had been scheduled in forty-eight hours. Landrum was lying on the table as we listened to the sound of her baby's heartbeat fill the room. A few minutes later, the technician returned and looked at the monitor. The heart rate appeared less like little mountains and more like chicken scratching. The baby was also either not moving consistently or not breathing properly. A nurse left the room to call Landrum's doctor. When she returned twenty minutes later, she gave us the news that the baby would be induced not later in the week but now. Both of us were terrified. "We need to call Latona," I told her.

An hour later, the doula arrived, wearing purple scrubs, her cloth bag filled with snacks, lavender lotion, and clary sage oil. She made sure the crayon-drawn affirmations were taped on the wall within Landrum's line of vision, then settled into a chair next to the bed, calm but watchful. Both of us were wearing "Team Simone" T-shirts my partner had made. A medical resident, who was white, like every single person who would attend Landrum throughout her labor and delivery, walked into the room with paperwork. Right away, she asked Landrum briskly, "Have you had any children before?"

"Yes, I've had three babies, but one died," Landrum explained warily, for the third time since she had been told she would need to be induced that day. Her voice was flat. "I had a stillbirth."

"The demise was last year?" asked the resident without looking up to see Landrum flinch at the word "demise."

"May I speak to you outside," Giwa said to the nurse caring for Landrum. In the hall she asked her to please make a note in the chart about the stillbirth for the parade of providers attending Landrum. "Each time she has to go over what happened, it brings her mind back to a place of fear and anxiety and loss," said Giwa later. "This is really serious. She's having a high-risk delivery, and I would hope that her care team would thoroughly review her chart before walking into her room."

Over the next ten hours, Giwa left Landrum's side only briefly. Several hours in, Landrum requested an epidural. According to hospital policy, no visitors can be in the room while an anesthesiologist administers it. When we returned about half an hour later, Landrum was angry and agitated, clenching her fists and talking much faster than usual. She had mistakenly been given a spinal dose of anesthesia—generally reserved for abdominal surgery—rather than the epidural dose used in childbirth. Now she had no feeling at all in her legs, and a splitting headache, which made her fearful that she had again developed preeclampsia. When she questioned the incorrect dose of anesthesia, Landrum told us that one of the nurses had said, "You ask a lot of questions, don't you?" and winked at another nurse in the room, then rolled her eyes. After Giwa questioned the nurse, she admitted the error.

As Landrum continued to loudly complain about what occurred, her blood pressure shot up, while the baby's heart rate dropped. Giwa glanced nervously at the monitor, the blinking lights reflecting off her face. She texted me, "Baby's not looking awesome right now. She needs to stay calm."

"What happened was wrong," Giwa said to Landrum, lowering her voice to a whisper and encouraging her to take deep breaths. "But for the sake of the baby, it's time to let it go."

She asked Landrum to close her eyes and imagine the color of her stress.

"Red," snapped Landrum, before finally laying her head on the pillow.

"What color is really soothing and relaxing?" asked Giwa, massaging her hand with lotion.

"Lavender," Landrum replied, taking a deep breath. Over the next ten minutes, Landrum's blood pressure dropped within normal range and the baby's heart rate stabilized.

At 1:00 a.m., a team of three young female residents bustled into the room; the labor and delivery nurse followed them, flipping on the overhead light. They were accompanied by an older man none of us had ever seen before. He briefly introduced himself as the attending physician. I was then shocked to see him plunge his hand between Landrum's legs to feel for the baby. We had been told that her ob-gyn might not deliver her infant, but a nurse had reassured us earlier in the day that if her doctor were not available, her doctor's husband, also an ob-gyn, would cover for her. This doctor, however, seemed a bit old to be the husband—and he wasn't—but no one explained the switch. Giwa raised an eyebrow and mouthed, "What's going on?" The Listening to Mothers III survey, a national sampling of twenty-four hundred women who gave birth between 2011 and 2012, found that more than a quarter of Black women meet their birth attendants for the first time during childbirth, compared with 18 percent of white women.

"He's ready," the doctor said, snapping off his gloves. "It's time to push."

One of the residents stepped forward and took his place, putting her hand into Landrum's vagina, feeling for the baby. Landrum gripped the side of the bed and closed her eyes, grimacing. The nurse, standing at her side, told Landrum, "Push! Now. You can do it." After about twenty minutes of pushing, the baby's head appeared. "This is it," the nurse told her. "You can do this," whispered Giwa on her other side. The nurse moved away, and I stepped in and held Landrum's hand.

Landrum bore down and pushed again. "You're doing amazing," said Giwa, not taking her eyes away from Landrum. The attending physician left the room to put on a clean gown. Landrum breathed in, closed her eyes, and pushed. More of the infant's head appeared, a slick cluster of black curls. The senior resident motioned to the third and most junior of the women, standing at her shoulder, and told her, "Here's your chance." The young resident took the baby's head and eased the slippery infant out. Though Landrum was oblivious to the procession of young residents taking turns between her legs without addressing her or looking her in the eye, or the fact that the attending physician wasn't in the room at all, I wasn't. It seemed like the height of disrespect. Landrum was now sobbing, shaking, laughing—all at the same time—flooded with the kind of hysterical relief a woman feels when a baby leaves her body and emerges into the world. A few minutes later, as she laid her hands across the baby's back, still coated with blood and amniotic fluid, Landrum told us she had decided to name him Kingston Blessed.

I stayed in New Orleans until the end of the week, leaving the hospital only to shower and sleep. Since I had been too frantic and nervous—while trying to appear calm—to take notes during Landrum's labor and delivery, as soon as I could, I spent about an hour writing down everything I remembered. I couldn't shake the way the residents, interns, doctor, and nurses had treated Landrum. Though these people had no idea that I was a journalist, I was still amazed that they were behaving so thoughtlessly in front of Giwa and me. It was also shocking that not one person of color was part of Landrum's medical team—in a hospital in New Orleans. That made me realize that they had absolutely no idea that anything they did was wrong. The sometimes subtle, other times heavy-handed ways that discrimination played out, exactly the way I had been reporting about it, was just business as usual.

After I went back to New York, I rewrote the story, now taking into account the week or so I had spent with Landrum before she went into labor and the scene in the delivery room. I also returned to New Orleans two months later to find Landrum settling into new motherhood with a cheerful, chunky Kingston. Giwa was still in the picture, making sure Landrum went to doctor appointments, giving advice about breast-feeding, and bringing the family food and supplies. For all of her work—before, during, and after the baby was born—Giwa was paid only $600.

In March 2002, the National Academy of Sciences, a private, nonprofit society of scholars, released a high-profile report documenting the unequivocal existence of racial bias in medical care, which many thought would mark a real turning point. *Unequal Treatment: Confronting Racial and Ethnic Disparities in Health Care* was so brutal and damning that it would seem impossible to turn away. The report, authored by a committee of mostly white medical educators, nurses, behavioral scientists, economists, health lawyers, sociologists, and policy experts, took an exhaustive plunge into more than 480 previous studies. Because of the knee-jerk tendency to assume that health disparities were the end result of differences in class, not race, they were careful to compare subjects with similar income and insurance coverage. The report found rampant, widespread racial bias, including that people of color were less likely to be given appropriate heart medications or to undergo bypass surgery or receive kidney dialysis or transplants. Several studies revealed significant racial differences in who receives appropriate cancer diagnostic tests and treatments, and people of color were also less likely to receive the most sophisticated treatments for HIV/AIDS. These inequities, the report concluded, contribute to higher death rates overall for Black people and other people of color and lower survival rates compared with whites suffering from comparable illnesses of similar severity. Though the report looked at disparities in health care between white Americans and minorities—African Americans, Native Americans, Hispanics, and several Asian subgroups—the Black-white gap was the most well documented and long-standing.

A mention of Dr. Kevin Schulman's 1999 experiment offered vindication of his work. "The real implication of the [Schulman] study was actually quite simple: doctors are human," wrote Thomas Perez, a civil rights attorney who contributed to *Unequal Treatment*. "Like lawyers, businesspeople, and other professionals, doctors are fallible and may discriminate, consciously or subconsciously . . . This study simply concluded that racial bias can affect who gets to the operating room."

The members of the committee of scientists and physicians who compiled *Unequal Treatment* were jolted by their own results, calling them both shocking and troubling. Black and other doctors and scientists of color were less surprised by what the report showed, since many had been shouting into the wind for years about the link between bias and racial health disparities. *Unequal Treatment* received widespread media attention. A *New York Times* editorial on March 22, 2002, was sharp in its rebuke. "To the extent that doctors are shaping their treatments based on subconscious biases or false stereotypes about how blacks or Hispanics will respond to their ailments or their treatments, the only lasting cure will be greater awareness and education for the medical profession, as the panel recommends," the *Times* editorial board wrote. "Unconscious racism is every bit as damaging as the more overt forms of bigotry."

A quotation by Goethe included in the first pages of the report would prove telling: "Knowing is not enough; we must apply. Willing is not enough; we must do." The report was not enough. Since its publication, hundreds more studies have examined the explicit link between racial discrimination and the physical and emotional health of Black people and other people of color, yet we've seen little forward movement on solutions.

When my story "Why America's Black Mothers and Babies Are in a Life-or-Death Crisis" was published in April 2018, I was thrilled by the widespread and largely positive response. Two weeks after the publication of the article, Governor Andrew M. Cuomo of New York announced a pilot program to expand Medicaid coverage for birth doulas, citing the need to target racial disparities in maternal mortality. His office explained that the story was instrumental in the decision. Inspired by the story, and by the Birthmark Doula Collective's work, the Women's Studies Department of Old Dominion University in Virginia launched a doula-training program as part of a service-learning requirement. When I visited the college in early 2020, ten students had been trained as doulas with a commitment to apply their skills to underserved populations in the Norfolk region.

Merck announced a commitment of an additional $10 million to support local initiatives addressing the racial disparity in maternal mortality in the United States. The piece was also a finalist for a National Magazine Award, the Oscars of our industry.

Most exciting for me, shortly after the publication of the piece, the State of Louisiana created the Perinatal Quality Collaborative to advance equity and improve birth outcomes in the state through the Safe Births Initiative. The organizers focused on a specific goal: to reduce severe maternal morbidity—near death—by 20 percent in women who, like Landrum, experience hemorrhage and/or severe hypertension/preeclampsia, in participating facilities. The facilities included both the hospital that employed the physician who ignored Landrum's repeated concerns and led to the death of Harmony and to Landrum's near death and the one where I observed her being treated so badly during the birth of Kingston. Those spearheading the project also hoped the work would narrow racial disparities in pregnancy outcomes.

But I was dismayed to receive dozens of negative comments from readers that were posted to the *Times* article or on Twitter or emailed to me directly. I know the evidence about the link between race, racism, and infant and maternal death is rock solid, and I offered a voluminous amount of it, including research on the role of toxic stress on the bodies of Black pregnant women, in a ten-thousand-word story—one of the longest ever run in the *Times* magazine. So I was surprised to receive aggressive notes marked by dismissal and denial, often fueled by explicit racism and drawing on racial stereotypes of Black women and the African American community. Readers, including health-care providers, called Landrum irresponsible, careless, and the victim of a dysfunctional culture. They accused her of lacking a healthy diet, which I never discussed and wasn't true. They blamed her for making poor lifestyle decisions, essentially holding her responsible for being beaten and abused by a violent partner.

By and large, I chose not to reply. Simone Landrum is a bright, kind person whom I respect and care about and who works hard to be a good mother to her three sons. She decided to allow me to attend her birth and tell her story because she wanted to make a difference and help other people. It takes courage to share your painful experiences in order to contribute to social change and help save the lives of other women and their children. For Landrum, trauma began early; she has had a very difficult life. She almost died as a child, narrowly escaping Katrina, which without a doubt was a tragedy that disproportionately affected African Americans and was not related to "poor decision making." She had to flee in water up to her chin; was that a choice? The dysfunction in this case was the choice of our government to abandon Black people in New Orleans and leave them to die. But no matter her circumstances, she deserved to be treated and cared for with respect and dignity by doctors and other health-care providers whose job it is to serve her.

Indeed, because I feared some people would judge Landrum and zero in on her disadvantaged background to explain away the loss of her baby, her near death, and her ill-treatment, I included the story of another Black woman whose legitimate concerns were ignored during the birth of her daughter, creating a harrowing and hectic near-death experience: Serena Williams. In January 2018, as I was putting the finishing touches on my article, the tennis champion shared the near-tragic story of the birth of her first child in *Vogue* magazine and on social media. In September 2017, the day after delivering her daughter, Alexis Olympia, via C-section in a hospital in Florida, Williams experienced a pulmonary embolism, the blockage of an artery in the lung by a blood clot. Though she had a history of this disorder, lived in fear of blood clots, understood how to diagnose and treat them—and was gasping for breath—she says medical personnel disregarded her knowledge and ignored her persistent concerns.

Williams—who was accompanied by her husband, Alexis Ohanian, the tech entrepreneur who co-founded Reddit—should have been able to count on the most attentive health care in the world. Still, her medical team seems to have been unprepared to monitor her for complications after her cesarean, including blood clots, one of the most common side effects of C-sections. Even after she received treatment, her problems continued when coughing, triggered by the embolism, caused her C-section wound to rupture. When she returned to surgery, physicians discovered a large hematoma, or collection of blood, in her abdomen, caused by medication, which required more surgery. Williams, who as an elite athlete knows her body intimately and has a net worth of hundreds of millions of dollars, spent the first six weeks of her baby's life bedridden.

What happened to the tennis superstar provided a clear-cut case study of discrimination in health care based on race—not class. In the next chapter I ask whether Landrum and Williams were vulnerable even before they set foot in a medical facility. Is something else about being Black bad for a woman's body and her baby?

CHAPTER FOUR

SOMETHING ABOUT BEING BLACK IS BAD FOR YOUR BODY AND YOUR BABY

This is the story of two women, a mother and her daughter, and two births over two generations. One mother was raised with a dozen other children by her grandmother who scratched out a living in rural Jamaica. The other, her daughter, grew up in a wealthy zip code in Southern California and attended private school, an elite college, and a top-ranked medical school before becoming a physician. One mother gave birth, easy as a finger snap, in a Black community at a hospital that has since been closed. The other's child was born in a facility affiliated with the renowned Cedars-Sinai, and the birth almost ended in tragedy. Their experiences support the findings of the Chicago-based neonatologists Richard David, MD, and James Collins, MD, who, over two generations, studied the birth weights of babies of hundreds of thousands of U.S.-born Black women, comparing them with the babies of Black women who had emigrated from some of the poorest countries in Africa and the Caribbean.

In the end, Dr. David concluded, "Something about growing up in America seems to be bad for your baby's birth weight."

The first mother was Avril Francis, an immigrant from the St. Andrew Parish just north of Kingston in Jamaica. In the 1950s, she grew up on a farm with her eleven cousins and two sisters, raised by their grandmother Lena, herself an immigrant from Panama. Lena cared for the houseful of children on the funds their parents sent home to support the boys and girls they had entrusted her with when they left the island to seek better lives. There were times when Avril and her cousins went to bed hungry or when she cut holes in the toes of shoes to make them last another few months. Avril finished high school and then managed to find her way to New York City, where she worked as a domestic and a nanny. Eventually, she realized her American dream—marriage to her high school sweetheart, Lennox Miller, an Olympic sprinter also from Jamaica, who had come to the United States to run track at the University of Southern California. In 1967, Avril and Lennox Miller settled in Altadena, a pastoral, upper-middle-class community in Southern California at the foot of the San Gabriel Mountains. When they bought their home on the mostly white East Side of town, they became the first Black family on their block. In 1971, while working as a flight attendant for TWA, Avril became pregnant with her first daughter, Inger, and again, four years later, with Heather. The young couple didn't have much money, so she wasn't able to afford the full complement of prenatal appointments, but both of her pregnancies, as well as the labor and deliveries, were free from complications. The older daughter, Inger, was born at normal birth weight and would go on to be an Olympic sprinter, like her father. Her younger sister, Heather, weighed a healthy seven and a half pounds at birth in 1976.

Nearly four decades later, Heather was living her mother's dream for her. A graduate of an elite private high school, Stanford University, and USC Medical School, she had become a physician and practiced not far from where she was raised. In 2014, she was married to a college professor and pregnant with her second child. As an ob-gyn, the daughter of an elite runner, and a high school and college athlete herself, Heather knew how to take care of her body; she did everything right. She stuck to a strict schedule of prenatal visits, ate healthfully, and took a cocktail of vitamins. She had planned to have a scheduled C-section, the baby delivered by a physician friend, with her husband and mother by her side.

Then, in her third trimester, Heather couldn't feel her infant moving. As she advised her patients, she lay on her side, had a snack, drank some water, and waited to feel her baby kick. If she really concentrated, Heather could feel the infant inside, but only faintly. She visited a high-risk specialist who told her the baby was small for her gestational age and ordered weekly monitoring. But toward thirty-eight weeks, Heather's gut told her something was wrong with her baby. If this child doesn't come out of my body, she thought, I'm going to have a demise. She was so terrified that her baby's heart would stop beating that she insisted on an induction; if she wasn't induced immediately, she told her doctor, she would induce herself. On October 14, Heather delivered Naia, weighing five pounds twelve ounces, almost two pounds less than she herself had been at birth. While technically a few ounces over the official classification for low birth weight, Naia was small for her gestational age and not out of the woods; she experienced neonatal hypoglycemia, sometimes found in preterm and small babies. Low blood sugar in the first few days after birth raises the risk of neurological damage, including to the brain. In her early years of life, Naia was slow to meet most of her growth and developmental milestones and also had problems sleeping and eating. She had allergic reactions to most of the normal food babies consume, sometimes life-threatening ones. Eventually, she was diagnosed with eosinophilic esophagitis, a chronic condition that causes inflammation of the esophagus. Six years old when I spoke to her mom, she is a sweet little girl who is both playful and a fighter. She loves animals and adores her big brother, Jaden, but is also tiny for her age. She takes medication to control her condition, avoids foods that kick up her allergies, and works with a therapist to help with delayed speech.

On the face of it, this outcome would seem unexpected. Though many factors come into play when it comes to individual births, education, wealth, healthy lifestyle, and quality prenatal and obstetric care are associated with infants born on time and at normal birth weight. Bigger babies generally signal robust health, while low-birth-weight infants are more likely to die in the first year of life. Conventional wisdom has it that the middle-class upbringing, education, and wealth that her immigrant mother struggled to create for Heather should have protected daughter and granddaughter from the kind of troubled birth outcome that Avril herself managed to avoid. Our country, the richest in the world, is an international leader in newborn intensive care, spending an estimated $26 billion a year to save babies born small and early. In general, in the United States health-care costs eat up 17 percent of our gross national product. Health-care expenditures account for only 6 percent of the GNP for Jamaica, where medical technology and innovation lag. America spends nearly $11,000 per person for health care compared with $320 in Jamaica. Money may buy good health care, but when you're Black in America, it cannot buy good health.

While the case of one mother-daughter pair is just that—a case study—their experiences sync up with the thousands of cases examined by Drs. David and Collins. Beginning in the 1990s, the two neonatologists set out to unravel the mystery of why in America Black infants are more than twice as likely as white babies to die before reaching their first birthdays. At the time, the high rate of infant mortality in Black women was widely believed by almost everyone, including doctors and public health experts, to affect *only* poor, less educated women who do have disproportionate numbers of lost babies. The underlying assumption was that poor Black teen moms had driven up rates of preterm and low-birth-weight babies, leading to increasing numbers of infant deaths. However, when the research pair analyzed the records of more than 100,000 births in Chicago between 1982 and 1983, they found that while income and education offered some protection, babies of more educated, higher-income Black parents were still more likely to be born small compared with their white counterparts.

Next, they wondered if the problem could be related to genetics: Could a preterm birth or low-birth-weight gene be the reason? If a defect in the Black body was causing infants to be born small, then women from the West African countries where the ancestors of African American women had been captured should have a similar problem of small babies. What's more, if the problem was produced by an inherited racial trait, shouldn't it be less pronounced in Black American women, who, as a population, had more European ancestry than their African-born counterparts? To test their theory, Drs. David and Collins examined the records of tens of thousands of babies born in Illinois between 1980 and 1995, homing in on three groups of women: U.S.-born Blacks, African-born Blacks, and U.S.-born whites. In their 1997 study, published in *The New England Journal of Medicine,* they found that the infants of the immigrant women from Africa were closely matched in size to the white, not the Black, U.S.-born babies. In other words, despite the disadvantages they experienced by being brought up in poorer, less developed nations, their newborns were larger and more likely to be full term than babies born to African American women. In 2002, the research pair and their colleague Shou-Yien Wu, MD, revisited the mystery of racial disparities in infant mortality. This time around they dismissed the preterm gene theory and were also careful to note that age, education, marital status, income, cigarette smoking, and the interval between pregnancies fail to account for African American infants' birth-weight disadvantage. For this study, published in the *American Journal of Epidemiology,* Drs. David and Collins looked at the birth records of infants born in Illinois between 1989 and 1991, along with those of their mothers who were born between 1956 and 1975—a total of approximately 328,000 infants. The researchers added two more groups of women along with their mothers: white immigrant mothers from Europe and Black moms from the Caribbean. To their surprise, the grandchildren of the Caribbean and African immigrant women were born smaller than their mothers had been at birth. The bottom line: the Black immigrant women's grandchildren were more likely to be small, just like African American babies. In contrast, once the daughters of white immigrant women became "Americanized," the weight of their infants shifted upward.

Finally, in 2007, Drs. David and Collins combined their previous studies into one deep dive that appeared in the *American Journal of Public Health.* For this study, they not only considered the effects of race but also looked at the more provocative question of what impact racism had on Black mothers and their babies. The pair spoke with Black women who had babies with normal weights at birth, comparing them with those whose babies were born under three pounds. They asked the mothers if they had ever been treated unfairly because of their race when looking for a job, in an educational setting, or in other situations. Those who experienced discrimination had a twofold increase in low birth weights. For those who reported discrimination in all three areas, the increase was nearly threefold. The researchers' conclusion: low birth weights among African American women have more to do with the experience of racism than with race.

I first began thinking about the Black-white disparity in preterm birth, low birth weight, and infant mortality as the health editor of *Essence* magazine from the late 1980s to the mid-1990s. At the time, I followed the conventional wisdom: that only poor women who lacked knowledge experienced tragic birth outcomes. This reflexive explanation for the death of a baby boiled down to blaming the mother, particularly if she was poor and Black. Was she eating badly, smoking, drinking, using drugs, not taking prenatal vitamins or getting enough rest, afraid to be proactive during prenatal visits, skipping them altogether, too young, or unmarried?

I covered the issue of infant mortality by encouraging the *Essence* audience of millions of mostly middle-class Black women readers to avoid unwanted pregnancy by taking control of their bodies—through birth control and sexual self-empowerment. We reminded them to pay attention to their health habits during pregnancy and make sure newborns slept on their backs. We urged readers to encourage teenagers in their orbit to just say no to sex and educate all the other women in their lives about the importance of prenatal care and healthy habits during pregnancy. This advice wasn't wrong, but it wasn't enough.

I revised my thinking in the early 1990s when a piece of research shook my core belief that we could educate our way out of the problem of poor birth outcomes plaguing Black America. In 1992, in a health policy class at the Harvard T. H. Chan School of Public Health, where I was a health communications fellow, my professor

Robert Blendon handed me the latest issue of *The New England Journal of Medicine*. Knowing I was the health editor of *Essence*, he said, "I thought you'd be interested in this." It contained what is now considered the watershed study on race, class, and infant mortality, unique because it isolated race in itself as a risk factor for poor birth outcomes. The study, conducted by four researchers at the Centers for Disease Control (CDC)—Kenneth Schoendorf, Carol Hogue, Joel Kleinman, and Diane Rowley—mined a database of close to a million previously unavailable linked birth and death certificates and found that infants born to college-educated Black parents were twice as likely to die as infants born of similarly educated white parents. In 75 percent of the cases, low birth weight was to blame. I was confused and so skeptical that I peppered Blendon with the kinds of questions about medical research that he encouraged us to ask in his course. Mainly I wanted to know *why* educated Black parents who could afford health care were experiencing this issue. "No one knows," he told me, "but this might have something to do with stress."

In 1996, I became pregnant, and the research became all too real for me. At the time, I had been promoted from health editor of *Essence* to executive editor, the success of my book *Body & Soul* continued, and I had a contract to co-write a self-help book aimed at Black parents. Without a doubt, I was a role model for Black women's health and wellness. Because I was in the public eye—and lecturing others in print and in person about the importance of health education and taking care of yourself—I was extremely careful to practice what I was preaching. I exercised nearly every day, adhered to a low-fat, high-vegetable diet, drank a lot of water, and saw my doctor once a year for a medical checkup and tests. So, it came as a total shock that though I had been doing everything right, something went wrong in the early months of my pregnancy. First I had a near miscarriage, and my doctor—a Park Avenue ob-gyn and female friend whom I trusted implicitly—put me on bed rest. After that first crisis was averted, she discovered that like Naia, Heather Miller's baby, my baby was far smaller than her gestational age would predict, even though I was in excellent health. My ob-gyn sent me to a specialist, where I was diagnosed with a condition called intrauterine growth restriction (IUGR), generally associated with mothers who have diabetes, high blood pressure, malnutrition, or infections including syphilis, none of which applied to me. During an appointment with a perinatologist—covered by my excellent health insurance—I was hounded with questions about my "lifestyle" and whether I drank, smoked, or used a vast assortment of illegal drugs. I wondered, "Does this doctor think I'm sucking on a crack pipe the second I leave the office?" In the absence of a medical condition, IUGR is almost exclusively linked with mothers who smoke or abuse drugs and alcohol. As my pregnancy progressed, but my baby didn't grow, my doctor decided to induce labor just short of one month before my due date, believing the baby would be healthier outside my body. My daughter was tiny, born at four pounds thirteen ounces, classified as low birth weight. Though she would grow to be a bright, athletic, healthy young woman, I thought back to Blendon's suggestion—that the less than healthy environment inside my uterus that had endangered my baby's life might have had something to do with stress. Had my own lived experience as a Black woman in America been bad for her birth weight?

In the mid-1990s, I was part of a study and its advisory board that hoped to answer this question. A team of female researchers from Boston and Georgetown Universities had noticed that most large, long-term medical investigations of women's health overwhelmingly comprised white women, so they launched the Black Women's Health Study (BWHS). The investigators contacted me at *Essence* to help recruit subjects, and I also signed on as one of fifty-nine thousand participants. They were interested in looking at a large group of Black women over time, taking the approach of the Nurses' Health Study. That long-term investigation, conducted by researchers from Harvard Medical School and other institutions and funded by the National Institutes of Health, began in 1976 and examined 120,000 educated, largely healthy women with access to medical care. However, the study's pool of subjects lacked diversity; the first cohort of nurses was 97 percent white.

Not long after the Black Women's Health Study launched, what happened to one research team member altered the course of the investigation. In 1995 several of the study's researchers became pregnant, but only one of them had a crisis: an African American doctoral student working as a research coordinator. She had a preterm birth that landed her baby in the neonatal intensive care unit (NICU). Though she had been healthy throughout her pregnancy, at thirty-four weeks her water broke unexpectedly. Hours after her baby's birth, his breathing became labored, and he required a ventilator for forty-eight hours and a feeding tube for six days during his ten-day stay in the NICU.

Julie Palmer, ScD, the principal investigator of the study, and her colleagues wondered why a healthy, middle-class, well-educated Black woman had a preterm birth when no one else in the group did and decided to examine the health effects of not just race but racism. In 1997, study investigators added several questions about everyday race-related insults, based on a scale created by David Williams, PhD, a prolific scholar in the area of racial health disparities. Those completing the scale are asked to check yes or no to the following statements:

1. You are treated with less courtesy than other people are.
2. You are treated with less respect than other people are.
3. You receive poorer service than other people at restaurants or stores.
4. People act as if they think you are not smart.
5. People act as if they are afraid of you.
6. People act as if they think you are dishonest.
7. People act as if they're better than you are.
8. You are called names or insulted.
9. You are threatened or harassed.

Williams, the Florence Sprague Norman and Laura Smart Norman Professor of Public Health and chair in the Department of Social and Behavioral Sciences at the Harvard T. H. Chan School of Public Health, created this set of questions in 1995, basically on a dare, after having been told that there was no way to measure racism. His scale has now been universally accepted, and also adapted and amended and used all over the world to measure the ways in which discrimination hurts health and shortens lives. Like many researchers in the area of health disparities, Williams has been beating the same drum for decades about race and health: that yes, as far as health goes, socioeconomic status and education matter, but they are not the whole story. The lived experience of being Black in America, regardless of income and education, also affects health.

I met Williams at a dinner in 2018 and spent the entire night talking to him, enthralled by his ideas, which were so similar to mine. He shared his thoughts about health inequality not in academic-speak but in plain English, soaked with the musical lilt of an upbringing on the Caribbean island of St. Lucia. The next day I googled him and read his scientific paper "Miles to Go Before We Sleep," a master class in the topic of racial inequities in health, complete with a hundred studies in the footnotes, many of them his own. Williams believed that big-ticket questions about discrimination at work, in housing, and by banks and the police, while obviously important, didn't go deep enough. So he added the other set of questions about the steady, soul-crushing experience of everyday racism, sometimes called microaggressions.

Several months after meeting Williams, I attended the American Public Health Association conference in San Diego to hear him deliver an eloquent keynote on health inequality and disparities and the responsibility of medical providers and public health practitioners to do something about this problem. Addressing the audience of thirteen thousand attendees, he was less comforting than he had been at the dinner and more insistent, sounding like a Baptist preacher and making good use of the divinity degree he had earned years earlier. To shatter the notion of the poverty explanation for health disparities, Williams explained, "In America, whites with only a high school education live longer than Blacks with a college degree or more," and illustrated his point with the shattering story of Clyde Murphy, a Black striver in the Yale class of 1970 who went on to earn a law degree from Columbia. Murphy became a top civil rights lawyer, but in 2010 died prematurely, at the age of sixty-two, from a blood clot in his lung. Murphy wasn't alone. In 2011, writing in the *Yale Alumni Magazine,* Ron Howell, Murphy's classmate, noted that forty-one years after their graduation, nine of thirty-two Black men who entered Yale in 1966 were dead, a death rate three times higher than that of the class as a whole. Williams offered a sliver of hope and a broad set of suggestions to attack the problem. Even as he spoke of that sliver, I couldn't shake the thought of the deaths of those Black men from Yale.

The researchers from the Black Women's Health Study used Williams's scale and also included three questions about institutional discrimination: Have you ever been treated unfairly due to your race at work, in housing, or by the police? When I filled out my survey, I answered yes to six out of the nine everyday insults and two of the three more hard-core examples of bias. In the end, BWHS research showed higher levels of diabetes, obesity, asthma, and preterm birth among women who reported the greatest experiences of racism.

When I first talked to Heather Miller, I was struck by our similar backgrounds—daughters of high-achieving Black mothers, hers from the Caribbean, mine from the South Side of Chicago, who had managed to overcome disadvantaged upbringings. Each of them sought better lives for their daughters, raising us in white suburban communities, which they understood offered opportunities that they didn't have. Like Miller's, my family integrated our neighborhood, and I was one of the only Black children in my elementary school, middle school, and high school. We both attended predominantly white universities and have spent most of our lives navigating white environments where we have lived and worked. Still, the trappings of the middle class weren't enough to protect us from the slow-burn damage of racism.

I felt a familiar sting as she described the experiences of her child-hood and early adulthood. As a young immigrant Black couple in a predominantly white environment, her parents were outsiders. Heather Miller attended the Westridge School for Girls in Pasadena. Though she remembers receiving an exceptional education, she was also the only Black girl in her class the entire nine years she attended, from fourth to twelfth grade. She rarely felt attractive. Miller was brown-skinned, fairly tall, and thin, but she also had curves—a round bottom and breasts—that stood out in a sea of thin white girls with long, straight hair, the mainstream look of the 1980s and 1990s. Her otherness was unambiguous and a source of curiosity. Girls kept up a steady stream of questions about her Jamaican par-ents, her skin color, and, of course, her hair. "Can I touch it?" she was asked constantly.

Miller was a rule-following, straight-A student who enjoyed read-ing and writing and was strong in science and math. She did her best to work hard in school, fly under the radar, and avoid either stick-ing out or disappointing her strict parents. But as she grew older, the slights from her classmates turned from innocent to hostile. She applied to Stanford and was accepted on the basis of her grades, col-lege entrance test scores, and athleticism. Still, she recalls peers and their parents who insisted that she only got in because she was Black. "You're lucky," a classmate said to her, "you're Black, so you'll be able to get in wherever you want." Another told her, "You don't have to worry; you've got affirmative action." At Stanford, Miller studied psychology but fulfilled her science requirements with an eye on medical school. She was almost dissuaded from pursuing medicine after an adviser told her she probably wasn't smart enough to be premed. In med school at the University of Southern California, the aggressions turned from micro to macro. Some of the instructors and attendings made it clear that neither Black students nor Black doctors were as smart as their white peers. Miller remembers sitting in the cafeteria with a group of her white classmates and an attend-ing pointing out that the only reason the dozen Black students—out of two hundred in the class of 2003—had made it to med school was affirmative action. The feeling of invisibility and erasure was stark and the pressure immense. She felt terrified of making any mistake, because she would never be given the benefit of the doubt.

Though she considered pediatrics, ultimately Miller chose ob-gyn. During her four-year residency between 2003 and 2007, she was attacked with a toxic mix of racism and sexism. She calls the program malignant. "If you were a woman who wasn't traditionally feminine, a person of color, [or] spoke with an accent, the mainly older white men who ran the residency treated you horribly," she recalls.

Over the years, she has been part of several ob-gyn practices, all but one time as the only Black person and sometimes the only woman; the Association of American Medical Colleges reports that only about 2.6 percent of physicians are Black women. In her current practice in Minneapolis, where she is still the only Black doctor, but one of several women, and where there is a diverse pool of patients, the slights continue to grate. Beginning in the early years of her medical career, she knew always to wear her white coat and introduce herself as Dr. Miller, to lock in her legitimacy. Otherwise, patients and even colleagues would assume she was a nurse or receptionist. Even after identifying herself as Dr. Miller and spending half an hour examining a patient and discussing a procedure, a patient might ask, "When will I talk to a doctor?" Or, "Who's doing the surgery?" Other times, after completing her rounds, a patient would complain, "I never saw a doctor."

Miller pauses after going through the inventory of mistreatment and listing the insults. She describes the pain of being undervalued and erased, and the isolation of a lifetime of being an "only," often forced to represent the entire race in all-white spaces. "Sometimes, I would know that something wasn't right or that I was being mistreated," she says. "But I had so few people to share it with. When you try and explain it to someone who doesn't understand what you're going through, they tell you you're being sensitive, or imagining it or making it racial. It's very confusing and isolating to not have people around who allow you to feel yourself or comfortable in your own skin." That constant vigilance, coping, and suppressed anger takes a toll. For Miller, stress manifests itself as splitting headaches that throb hard and hot and crushing exhaustion. She describes the feeling as wearing; I immediately think of weathering.

Research conducted by Drs. David and Collins as well as the investigators behind the Black Women's Health Study has shown that something about being a Black woman in America is bad for her body and her baby. Taking it a step further, Arline Geronimus, a professor at the University of Michigan School of Public Health, provides the best current explanation of how lived experiences can become biology. Her concept of weathering explains that high-effort coping from fighting against racism leads to chronic stress that can trigger premature aging and poor health outcomes. It works this way: stress, the body's response to a perceived threat, prompts the brain to release hormones, including adrenaline and cortisol. This, in turn, causes blood pressure to increase and the heart rate to speed up. Short, infrequent bursts of this fight-or-flight response are normal, but when it happens again and again, it can turn deadly, eroding health and accelerating aging. Also, as the stressors pile up and feed on each other, they can lead to unhealthy coping mechanisms—drinking, smoking, poor food choices, and drug use. Those who are economically disadvantaged have added stressors in their day-to-day fight for survival, but even educated, well-off African Americans struggle with anger and grief triggered by everyday racist insults and microaggressions. These can, over time, deteriorate the systems of the body.

Geronimus, who coined the term "weathering," chose this metaphor, leaning into its double meaning. To weather means to wear down, but it also means to withstand, as in weathering a storm. Though discrimination and bias wear away the bodies of those who must continually beat them back, she notes that the positive forces of family, friendship, and community support can help a person withstand, resist, and undo the negative effects. And while chronic stress interferes with the health of an average person, it can upend a pregnant person. Pregnancy is already a stress test for the body, and the added and cumulative strain of fighting against racial bias and discrimination, and its weathering effect, far too often turns what should be the happiest day of a woman's life into tragedy or near tragedy. Black women, more frequently than other women, enter pregnancy with health disadvantages; studies have found that disproportionate numbers of African American women of childbearing age, in their twenties and early thirties, already suffer from chronic diseases, including high blood pressure, that show up in other Americans later in life. Though the vast number of Black women have healthy pregnancies and babies, Geronimus and others believe that the cumulative impact of battling back racism drives up their risk of preterm birth, low birth weight, and infant and maternal death.

This idea first intrigued Geronimus and provided the seeds of her weathering research more than four decades ago. In the fall of 1976, Geronimus, an undergraduate at Princeton University, was straddling two worlds. A political theory major, she worked as a research assistant to Charles Westoff, who studied teen pregnancy, and she also volunteered at a Planned Parenthood alternative school for pregnant girls in Trenton, one of New Jersey's poorest cities, where she mingled with real-life examples of her professor's research. Her Princeton professors believed that teen pregnancy was at the root of inner-city poverty and a major cause of poor health in Black America. Helping young Black girls understand the dire consequences of teen pregnancy and teaching them how to avoid it, they insisted, would turn around poverty and health trends and prevent the problem of "babies having babies." But spending time with girls at the alternative school showed Geronimus something else. The girls weren't losing out on higher education, careers, and other opportunities as a result of pregnancy. Those advantages didn't exist in their communities. Plus, getting pregnant wasn't necessarily a drag on the young women; many of them were experienced with raising children, having helped care for siblings and other family members. Inspired by the book *All Our Kin,* the anthropologist Carol B. Stack's ethnography of three years in a low-income Black community, Geronimus understood that many of the young women lived in a warm embrace of family and community support, or kin, in stark contrast to the popular image of the "ghetto" as deficient and dysfunctional. She started to see that societal barriers, inequality, and lack of choices, not teen pregnancy, were the origin of the socioeconomic problems the Black community was struggling against.

After Princeton, Geronimus attended the Harvard School of Public Health, where she wrote her dissertation on the association between maternal age and pregnancy outcomes. In white women she found that infant mortality was highest among teen mothers, but she was surprised that the opposite was true for Black women: Black teenage mothers had lower infant death rates than Black mothers in their twenties. Using infant health as a proxy for maternal health, Geronimus's data suggested that the average Black woman might be less healthy at twenty-five than at fifteen, meaning that something was taking a toll on her body as her birthdays passed.

In 1987, Geronimus landed at the University of Michigan, where she continued her research in infant mortality, race, and maternal age. That year, in the journal *Population and Development Review,* read by few outside the social science world, she pointed out again that slightly older Black women had higher rates of infant death than teenage girls, presumably because they were older and stress had more time to wear down their bodies. Her published work contradicted the widely accepted notion that teenage girls were to blame for high rates of Black infant mortality. In 1990, at a meeting of the American Association for the Advancement of Science, Geronimus presented research showing that teen mothers' socioeconomic outcomes were no worse than those of older moms. Often, pregnancy gave young women access to programs like Medicaid, or they created ties with the families of the fathers of their children, which improved their economic position. Geronimus's goal was to shift the focus from teen pregnancy to the root causes of poverty and disadvantage in urban areas. But the period was marked by a political and culture war over family planning and abortion rights, and the backlash was swift. Karen Pittman, a Black sociologist, attacked Geronimus in *The New York Times.* "Her facts are misrepresentative, her premise is

wrong, and the policy implications of her arguments are perverse,"
said Pittman, who had recently launched an adolescent pregnancy
prevention initiative for the Children's Defense Fund. Geronimus
recalls that in another publication, a headline screamed, "Research
Queen Says Let Them Have Babies." Geronimus was criticized by
colleagues and even received anonymous death threats at her office
in Ann Arbor and at home. She remembers that at the time there
were more calls to the University of Michigan to complain about
her, to demand she be fired, than about anybody in the history of
the university.

Geronimus persisted, and in a 1992 study in the journal *Ethnicity
and Disease,* she introduced her weathering hypothesis to explain
why the health of African American women may begin to deteriorate in early adulthood: as a physical consequence of cumulative disadvantage. In subsequent years, she honed and shaped her theory,
drawing on the scholarship of her former University of Michigan
colleague Sherman James. He had come up with the concept of John
Henryism to describe how battling against racism deteriorates the
systems of the body, using the folk hero John Henry as a metaphor.
According to the legend, Henry, a steel-driving railroad worker, won
an epic battle of strength against a mechanical steam drill but died
from total emotional and physical depletion after the victory. A folk
song describes his agonizing story: "He worked so hard, it broke
his heart. John Henry laid down his hammer and died, Lord, Lord,
John Henry laid down his hammer and died." His high-effort striv-
ing had killed him. James's scholarship led Geronimus to understand
that it was more than stress as a response to insults that caused harm
to the body; it was the relentless effort in the face of discrimination
and inequality. Or, as the saying about being Black in America goes,
having to work twice as hard for half as much.

Still, at that point Geronimus didn't have a biological explanation for how stress or effort led to illness. She found direction in the
research of Bruce McEwen, a neuroendocrinologist at Rockefeller
University who had studied the effects of environmental and psychological stress on the body. He had coined the term "allostatic

load," which is measured using a set of biomarkers that become disrupted when the body releases hormones in the face of sustained stress. The biomarkers include blood pressure, heart rate, cholesterol, and body mass index. For her 2006 study, published in the *American Journal of Public Health,* Geronimus and her team used data collected via a questionnaire on various health and social factors and a clinical examination during which measurements of height, weight, and blood pressure were taken and blood drawn. They found that because of the double jeopardy of being Black and female in America, Black women suffered the highest allostatic load scores, compared with Black men or with white men or women. These differences, they wrote, were not explained by poverty. Well-off Blacks had higher scores than did poor whites. Now Geronimus was able to explain how the stress associated with racism weathers the body at the biological level.

Heather Miller, her husband, her son, and her mother, Avril, who has relocated to Minneapolis, love little Naia fiercely and are doing everything they can as a family to correct what happened to her at birth. Heather learned from her immigrant parents not to complain, not to look back, not to blame others, not to be weighed down by regret, but instead to put her head down, work relentlessly, and soldier ahead. But Miller does wonder, as I do, if something about being a Black woman in America affected her body and her baby.

Like Heather Miller, U-Meleni Mhlaba-Adebo is the daughter of an immigrant mother from a disadvantaged country and the mother of an African American child whose birth in the United States almost ended in tragedy. But as a poet and performance artist, U-Meleni, unlike Miller, races toward her emotions and has expressed in her work some of the hardest truths about the lived experience of being a Black woman in America and a daughter of immigrant Africans. I used her poem "Breaking Point," from her 2016 book, *Soul Psalms,* to describe the ache.

Helen Murapa, U-Meleni's mother, was born and raised on a farm in the Chipinge District of what was then called Southern Rhodesia. Now Zimbabwe, the country is one of the world's poorest, and life expectancy tops out at age sixty-one. During the 1950s and early 1960s, Helen's parents supported their five children by farming sweet potatoes, mangoes, pumpkins, and bananas and raising goats and cows on twelve acres of land. Beginning in Helen's teen years, her country was engulfed in societal unrest, often violent, as the Black majority battled against white rule. A few years after Helen was able to leave to study in the United States, civil war broke out. By 1974, when she became pregnant, Helen was living in Boston, married to a man from her country, pursuing her master's degree at Simmons College. Her daughter U-Meleni was born on November 9, 1974, healthy at eight pounds.

Helen divorced a few years after U-Meleni's birth and returned to Zimbabwe with her young daughter. U-Meleni attended boarding school in Zimbabwe and South Africa, before returning to Massachusetts for college in 1994. She attended Wentworth Institute of Technology, a small STEM-focused college where the majority of students were white men, before transferring to the University of Massachusetts in Boston to study social psychology. She lived with her father, stepmother, and half sisters, on an all-white block in suburban Newton. It took her a few years before she understood the full extent of living in America as a Black woman. She describes her early years in the United States as being wet behind the ears as far as racism went. But that ended. When she rode the subway, returning home to Newton, where less than 3 percent of residents are African American, people would ask her, "Where are you going? Why are you getting off here?" Another time, on her way back from shopping, she was accused of stealing groceries from an older white woman. The police sided with U-Meleni only after she showed them her receipt. Another time, her then boyfriend was falsely accused of stealing gas at a pump, but this time when the police came, they threatened to arrest him. After, she remembers, she felt lividly angry and mortified by the experience. "By then, I was starting to understand what was going on in this country." In 1998, just after graduation from college, while she was interviewing for a position at a bank, a white interviewer looked at her hair, which was neatly styled in Nubian knots, and asked her, "Could you maybe do something about your hair?" "My father had warned me that no one would hire me if I didn't straighten my hair, but I refused," she recalls, still angered by the experience. "Essentially this woman was saying be less Black." U-Meleni performed the following poem, "Have You Ever," as part of the Black Love project at the Castle of Our Skins concert and performance series in Roxbury, Massachusetts, in November 2020:

> Have you ever died
> While breathing
> While standing vacant
> Tsunami of tears
> Flood in your brain?
> Have you ever lost your voice
> From screaming
> between borders of reason and reality?
> Have you ever heard shallow breaths
> like earthquakes
> shaking the foundation
> that are your feet?
> Have you ever watched your foundation
> break in two continents
> Unable to split yourself into two?
> Have you ever cried in the arms of your shadow?
> Am tired of regurgitating names,
> tired of flowers,
> altars to the dead
> I can't breathe.
> These streets,
> This land,
> This country.
> This world.

Cemetery of black and brown bodies
Mine,
Always mine,
Always mine,
Ours

By 2000, U-Meleni had found a steady job as a teacher, where she was flooded with stories of the traumas and tragedies of her students and their parents. After work, she performed as a poet, singer, and storyteller. In 2009, she married her husband, Olumide, a Nigerian American, and the following year she was pregnant with their son. At age thirty-six, U-Meleni, who was a runner and in excellent physical condition, experienced her pregnancy as smooth and uneventful. She had crafted a birth plan, envisioning her son being born in a calm, "namaste kind of environment" at the Cambridge Birth Center. As her March 18, 2011, due date approached, she bought candles and chose music, Nina Simone and Jill Scott, and planned for her husband and mother to be with her during labor and delivery. Two days before her son was born, she threw a butterfly party to honor and celebrate fifteen women in her life, including her three sisters, and to ask for their offerings for her baby. Her sisters made a plaster cast of her belly, and her friends wrote messages to her son. She and Olumide decided to name him Jabulani, which means "to be happy." "The event was beautiful, really beautiful," she remembers. She wrote this piece on September 4, 2010:

Poem for Jabu

I dream of you though you are not yet born
I think of how you will look, smell, and feel
You are our love manifest growing inside my belly
Evidence that I don't yet see but feel in my heart
I wonder if you can hear us speak your name
Feel your father's touch

When he rubs my belly
Comforting us both
We are excited to be your parents
And we hope we are worthy
Of this blessed experience to watch you bloom
Amen

But the next day, still more than three weeks before her due date, U-Meleni had severe back pain and went to the birthing center to get checked. Immediately, they sent her across the street to Cambridge Hospital, where doctors discovered that her blood pressure was through the roof. She was diagnosed with preeclampsia and given magnesium, which, though she didn't know it, she was allergic to. Soon the situation had progressed to an emergency, and both mother and baby were in distress. U-Meleni and Olumide went in an ambulance from Cambridge Hospital to Tufts Children's Hospital, which had a state-of-the-art NICU. There, after several hours, the baby's heart rate dropped, and U-Meleni learned that her perfect birth plan had turned into a crisis. When she understood that her infant would be delivered via C-section, she describes the feeling as complete panic and shock. The process was worse than she imagined. "It felt like a Mack truck, maybe several of them, had had a complete accident on my uterus," she says. "And then like a chain saw came and shredded my stomach and yanked my baby out." The trauma left U-Meleni with low blood pressure and in unimaginable pain. When she finally felt better, she asked, "Where's my baby?" She was brought to the NICU and saw Jabulani, pale and tiny, just three pounds one ounce, and attached by wires to several machines. She was so jolted that she fainted. She was later told, like me, and like Heather Miller, that the baby inside her body had stopped growing, in her case at twenty-nine weeks. He stayed in the NICU for two weeks.

Ten years later, Jabulani is tall and athletic, with high cheekbones and chocolaty skin like his mother. His name fits him. U-Meleni has lived in America for more than half her life now and understands that something about living here is bad for her overall well-being. She describes the feeling best in her poem "Her Body Is a Weapon," from her album *Soul Psalms—Birth, Death, Resurrexion:*

Her body is a weapon,
covered with thorns
Her body is a weapon,
Numb, she feels pain no more
You see no one ever told her that she was beautiful
No one, no one ever told her that she looked like a queen
All they did was demean,
her body is a weapon
Bleak, cold and forlorn
Using her thighs as ammunition
Fighting a battle only pain could conceive
Wet red blood dripping in between her legs
Ruptured soul that she is
And they ask her to be brave
They ask her to believe that she's beautiful
When the ones who create her
Are the ones who enslave
Puncture her soul, rupture her body, massacre her core

CHAPTER FIVE

WHERE YOU LIVE MATTERS

Danielle Bailey grew up in Walnut Cove, North Carolina, a town of about fifteen hundred in Stokes County. As a child in the 1980s, she cherished warm, lazy weekends at Belews Lake—pronounced "Blues"—several miles from her home near Main Street. She recalled lounging on the tree-lined banks of the nearly four-thousand-acre lake and dipping into the blue-green water that shimmered when the sun hit the surface in just the right spots. Years later, after two semesters at North Carolina A&T, she returned home to marry her high school sweetheart, Tony Lash, pregnant with their first child. When the couple decided to buy a house to raise their son, Anthony, and their daughter, Amani, who was to come five years later, they chose a two-story, three-bedroom brick home on Pine Hall Road, not far from the lake Danielle had loved as a child. Living close to a body of water that provided recreation and pleasure and attracted people from the nearby counties on weekends for boating, fishing, and swimming to Danielle signaled prosperity.

These days fewer people gather at Belews Lake, especially on weekdays, when only one or two boats float lazily near the shore. At some sections of what is actually a reservoir, created in the 1970s to provide cooling waters for Duke Energy's Belews Creek Steam Station, the water is less fresh than turgid and tepid. On Saturdays, the parking lot at the recreational access entrance on Pine Hall Road is full of trucks with boat trailers in tow as their owners troll for spotted bass. Though a sign encourages fishing, most of these fishermen have no idea that between 1974, the year Duke Energy located one of the largest coal-fired electric generating plants in the state in tiny Walnut Cove, and 1986, nineteen species of fish were killed off by toxic wastewater released by the facility, according to a 2002 study by the U.S. Forest Service.

For many who, like the young Danielle Bailey, were drawn to the waters of Belews Lake, the stacks of the plant that loom in the near distance belching out thick white steam barely register. They do not know that the lake and the land around it might have sickened Danielle—and many of her neighbors. In 2014, the danger became glaringly apparent when a 324-acre pond containing coal ash, a toxic by-product of the plant laced with unsafe levels of lithium, radium, selenium, mercury, and other harmful substances, spilled into the lake after a 48-inch storm pipe burst. Belews Creek and the Dan River, which snake through Stokes County, were also contaminated. Because the pond was unlined, over time pollution also seeped into the soil and groundwater. Coal ash is also buried across the area in landfills, which look like gentle rolling hills. Though no one can prove it definitively, living in this toxic area, which Danielle Bailey-Lash called home for many years, might have led to her brain cancer.

Where you live matters. From birth to death, the conditions in the social and physical environment where people make their homes, work, attend school, play, and pray have a significant influence on health outcomes. Those in the public health field call these conditions social determinants of health. Living in safe communities, with adequate health-care services, outdoor space, clean air and water, public transportation, and affordable healthy food—as well as education, employment, and social support—contributes to longer, healthier lives. And the opposite is true: when residents lack a healthy environment and basic services and support, their lives are cut short. When I returned to the South Side of Chicago in 2020 to see where my Mississippi-born grandparents and their siblings settled during the Great Migration—and which my immediate family left in 1969—I could see the outsized effects of race and place on health.

In January 2020, my mother and I traveled to Chicago. While there, she wanted to show me her old stomping grounds, and we had a long list of locations to visit, most of them in the Englewood section. It included one of her childhood homes, the house she and my father had lived in shortly after their wedding, her elementary and high schools, and the elementary school I had attended before we moved to Denver. I was most excited to revisit Mr. Brice's, a liquor shop on Vernon Avenue owned by my dad's close friend. On Saturdays my father would stop in to hang out and talk about fishing with Mr. Brice, who would give my sister and me free candy and ice cream sandwiches. His store served as a welcoming kind of community center for the neighborhood. The oaky smell of any liquor store still brings back that memory.

But the working-class Black community we remembered with warmth and nostalgia was gone; we were shocked by the condition of Englewood and other South Side neighborhoods. My mother's childhood home had been razed, reduced to a garbage-filled vacant lot. The home she lived in with my father was boarded up, as was her elementary school, Betsy Ross. Mine, John Harvard Public School, was still there, now known as the Harvard School of Excellence, but the houses across the street were abandoned, as were several nearby business storefronts. Englewood High School, which my mom attended with the playwright Lorraine Hansberry, had been closed in 2008 due to poor performance. Mr. Brice's was long gone. I had expected gentrification, but this community of about twenty-four thousand residents—in the middle of the country's third-largest city—reminded me of the rural Mississippi my family had left behind. We later learned that Chicago has the country's widest racial disparity in life expectancy—a gap of thirty years between Streeterville (nine miles north), where people expect to live to ninety, and my mom's old neighborhood, Englewood, where people live to only age sixty.

Where they live also matters to the people of Walnut Cove, who are suffering under the weight of an inequity that can damage the health of a community: environmental injustice. From foul water in Flint, Michigan, to deadly chemicals that have poisoned a large corridor of Louisiana known as Cancer Alley, Black and poor communities shoulder a disproportionate burden of the nation's pollution, which has been well documented for decades, thanks to a pileup of evidence that scientists and policy makers began gathering beginning in the 1970s. A wide-ranging report from 2017 added to the stockpile of proof: "Fumes Across the Fence-Line," compiled by the NAACP and the Clean Air Task Force, showed that African Americans are 75 percent more likely than the average American to live in so-called fence-line communities. These are defined as areas near facilities that emit hazardous waste. Breathing air poisoned by emissions is the most direct, unavoidable consequence of life in a fence-line community, depriving residents of their most fundamental right, the right to breathe. Installing facilities that inflict negative health, social, and economic outcomes on communities that generally didn't want them has been called a new kind of Jim Crow.

In 2018, researchers from the Environmental Protection Agency (EPA) proved that though poverty matters as far as who is exposed to pollution, race plays an outsized role. A study conducted by the EPA's National Center for Environmental Assessment looked at facilities emitting air pollution, along with the racial and economic profiles of surrounding communities, and found that Black Americans are subjected to higher levels of air pollution than white Americans regardless of their wealth. The research, which was published in the *American Journal of Public Health,* noted that Black Americans are exposed to 1.54 times more of the kind of sooty pollution that comes from burning fossil fuels than the population at large. This dirty air is associated with lung disease, including asthma, as well as heart disease and premature death. Ironically, another study, published in 2019 in the *Proceedings of the National Academy of Sciences,* showed that despite disproportionate exposure to air pollution, Black and Latinx people are less likely than whites to consume the goods and services that produce it. For example, compared with white people, Black Americans are more frequently exposed to the emissions from plants and factories that produce fuel, though, per capita, they fly and drive less.

The urgency of this environmental crisis has been hastened by climate change. When a weather disaster strikes, people of color are hit first, worst, longest, and hardest. In December 2017, several months after Hurricane Harvey produced catastrophic flooding in Texas and other states, two scientists from the University of California, Berkeley, used government data to calculate that the record rainfall, which added up to fifty inches in some areas, was 38 percent higher than would be expected if the world were not growing warmer. Black and brown people shouldered the brunt of the disaster, which destroyed hundreds of thousands of homes and businesses and killed nearly one hundred people. Those in fence-line communities, already burdened by pollution from oil, gas, and chemical plants, faced a kind of double jeopardy when the wind and rains came.

Lowndes County, Alabama, provides a stark example of the ways climate change has amplified the severe effects of a long-standing environmental crisis. This historically Black community has for decades been contaminated by raw sewage resulting from an inadequate waste system. More recently, long, erratic rainy seasons and warmer temperatures triggered by climate change have created an emergence of hookworm in the community. When it rains, wastewater bubbles up into homes through sinks, tubs, and toilets, and puddles of sewage contaminated with human waste collect in the soil that gave the Black Belt states of the South their name. A 2017 survey by the Baylor College of Medicine found that more than one-third of Lowndes County residents tested positive for hookworm, a tropical disease associated with developing countries and long thought to be eradicated in the United States. Humans contract this intestinal parasite through dirt contaminated with feces. In 2017, a United Nations official toured the area and noted that the contamination was "very uncommon in the First World. It's not a sight that one normally sees." Tragically, Lowndes County is located along the route of the Reverend Martin Luther King Jr.'s historic 1965 Selma-to-Montgomery civil rights march—a symbol of pride and resistance.

In May 2010, Danielle Bailey-Lash, then thirty-five and with two young children at home, was working as an administrator for her mother, Sandra, who owned Sandy's Playschool, a day-care center not far from her daughter's home on Pine Hall Road. Danielle had been suffering from agonizing migraines for months, and pain medication provided little relief. Sometimes the pain was so intense that only walking around with an ice pack on her head as she went about her duties at the day-care center provided any relief. But on May 8, the pain rose to brain-splitting intensity. Sandra looked at her daughter, who was in so much pain that she could barely turn her head, and insisted, "Call Tony and have him take you to the emergency room." At the ER at what was then known as Forsyth Memorial Hospital, doctors discovered a tumor over Danielle's right ear the size of a baseball and admitted her right away. She was diagnosed with stage 3 glioblastoma, an aggressive form of brain cancer, and given three to six months to live. She required a craniotomy to remove part of her skull in order to take out the tumor. Her mother organized terrified family members into shifts so Danielle would never be alone in the hospital. She brought in the bishop of her church and gathered Danielle's husband, aunt, and uncle for prayer vigils at her bedside. Days after her surgery, drifting in and out of sleep, her head wrapped in bandages and swollen three times its normal size, Danielle told her mom not to be afraid. With a kind of otherworldly calm, she explained that God had spoken to her and Jesus had come into the room. "I am at peace, Mom," she said. "I am going to be fine." After a punishing round of chemotherapy and radiation treatments, the cancer eventually went into remission, and Danielle insisted that her friends and family stay positive about her condition and prognosis.

Almost four hundred miles north, in Washington, D.C., Caroline Armijo heard from a mutual friend that Danielle had had surgery.

Caroline and Danielle had known each other since they met in gym class in seventh grade at Southeastern Middle School in Walnut Cove. The bookish girls, one Black, the other white, got along right away. After graduation from South Stokes High School, they went their separate ways—Danielle to North Carolina A&T, a historically Black university, Caroline to the University of North Carolina, Chapel Hill. There, Caroline met her husband, Enrique, and in 2005 the couple moved to Washington, D.C., where he worked as a lawyer. She leaned into her artistic talents, and they started a family. When Caroline learned that Danielle's surgery was the result of a brain tumor, she was rattled. From her mother and others back home, she had begun hearing about so many friends, neighbors, and relatives diagnosed with cancer: her mom's cousin died of leukemia, the beloved director of a funeral home passed away from breast cancer, a childhood neighbor who loved to fish in Belews Lake died from a brain tumor, and his best friend also died from brain cancer. And now Danielle. Though cancer is an unpredictable disease that sometimes strikes without logic, she wondered why her friend, a young, healthy nonsmoker and nondrinker, would contract an aggressive form of brain cancer whose median age at diagnosis in the United States is sixty-four. Shaken, Caroline decided to look into what could be going on in their hometown. She befriended experts on the internet and read books and listened to podcasts about the environment. She had never heard of coal ash and googled "is coal ash toxic?" Eventually, she discovered a report from the environmental group Earthjustice, which had mounted an advocacy campaign, Coal Ash Contaminates Our Lives. She learned that each year in the United States, 140 million tons of coal ash pollution are produced by coal plants, with nearly 750 sites around the country storing some form of the substance. Seventy percent of coal ash ponds are located in poor communities, and nearly all of them have leaked into nearby water sources, according to EPA data, disgorging known environmental toxicants into the land and water. She also came to understand that North Carolina had more than one hundred coal ash disposal sites and that her friend Danielle and her family were living down the road from one.

By 2012, when Caroline returned to North Carolina with her husband and the first of their two children, settling in Greensboro, about forty-five minutes from Walnut Cove, she knew it was time to have a heart-to-heart with Danielle. By then, Caroline's first cousin had been diagnosed with a brain tumor, and his wife's best friend had passed away a year earlier from a brain tumor, one of four people in their social circle in their fifties who had died. Caroline didn't want to overwhelm Danielle, who had outlived her original doomsday prognosis and was struggling back from a second craniotomy, but she felt compelled to warn her that the poison from Duke Energy might be the cause of her cancer. The two friends emailed, and as gently as possible Caroline explained what she knew. Danielle remembered being in denial, unable to believe that the lake she loved could be harming her, that the company down the road could be poisoning the community with no remorse or retribution, and that the government could allow something like this to happen. But when Caroline eventually told her, "I wish you could move," she listened. A home inspection also shocked her into action: it found elevated levels of radon, a radioactive gas that can cause cancer, in her drinking water. Given the contamination, health officials advised her to avoid drinking, cooking with, or doing laundry with her tap water, and not to take showers for longer than a few minutes at a time. Two years later, the state would admit trying to cover up the extent of the crisis after a toxicologist working under the governor testified that state officials told residents their water was safe knowing it wasn't. Danielle thought of her daughter, Amani, born small and premature, playing on a tire swing and splashing into the waters of the lake. And of herself, and the cancer that was eating away her brain, and decided she had to get out.

In 2014, she and her daughter moved from the house on Pine Hall Road into Regency Apartments, a brick complex in the center of the town of Walnut Cove, miles away from the lake and plant.

She also forced herself to come to the difficult conclusion that something sinister was going on, and accompanied Caroline to a meeting of Appalachian Voices, an environmental justice organization that had been pressuring Duke Energy to clean up the local coal ash mess. Danielle, shy and trusting by nature, was not a natural activist. But a monumental crisis helped cement her decision to take her first steps into environmental advocacy: the same year Danielle left Pine Hall Road, another Duke Energy plant, downstream from Walnut Cove, spilled nearly forty thousand tons of coal ash and twenty-seven million gallons of wastewater into the Dan River. This event, which received national media attention, spiked her already burdened community with more toxic pollutants. Many local residents learned about the disaster from Facebook. At the same time, their feeds were flooded with prayers for a ten-year-old neighbor of Danielle's who had survived a brain tumor but was now fighting lung cancer.

Along with attending Appalachian Voices meetings, Danielle tried to sound the alarm in small ways. At one point, while waiting to go into treatment at the regional medical facility where she received cancer care, she saw two other people from her small town. When she mentioned the connection between herself, her neighbors, and the Duke plant to her health-care providers, she says they brushed her off. When she brought flyers about coal ash, pointed to a few more people from Walnut Cove undergoing cancer treatment at their center, and told them about her ten-year-old neighbor, they didn't believe her. Even when she brought her cancer specialists the home inspection that showed her water was tainted, they didn't take her seriously. Instead, she was referred to a nutritionist, who told her to avoid eating food from cans to prevent exposure to aluminum, which has no direct connection to brain cancer.

Black people have long been blamed for the health problems that plague them, with little acknowledgment of the condition of their communities. The centuries-old focus on genetic and physiological differences between Blacks and whites has masked the brutal effects of racial discrimination and structural inequality. In 1896, when African Americans were reeling and still recovering from the effects of 250 years of enslavement and struggling through the reactionary years of Jim Crow, Frederick L. Hoffman, a German immigrant and statistician for the Prudential Insurance Company of America, published *Race Traits and Tendencies of the American Negro.* His much-lauded report attributed poor health outcomes of African Americans to racial inferiority and genetic susceptibility—or, in his words, a "race proclivity to disease and death." The 330-page article, a mash-up of statistics, eugenic theory, observation, and speculation, was published in the then-prestigious journal *Publications of the American Economic Association* and used statistical data to deny Black Americans life insurance. *Race Traits* remained the gold standard for evidence-based statistical research into race and health for years. It supported the myth that Black Americans died because they were inferior, and they were inferior because they died. "It is not in the conditions of life," Hoffman wrote, "but in the race traits and tendencies that we find the causes of excessive mortality."

To counter Hoffman, the eminent Black sociologist W. E. B. Du Bois undertook his own investigation into the health conditions and high mortality rates of Blacks and made a point of highlighting the social conditions that Hoffman had so studiously ignored. Du Bois and his team did extensive shoe-leather fieldwork that he would turn into his 1899 opus, *The Philadelphia Negro,* canvassing neighborhoods and interviewing residents in twenty-five hundred households. In a later work, *The Health and Physique of the Negro American,* Du Bois wrote, "With the improved sanitary condition, improved education and better economic opportunities, the mortality of the race may and probably will steadily decrease until it becomes normal." Du Bois was unsparing on the lack of compassion for the health and well-being of Black Americans. "The most difficult social problem in the matter of Negro health is the peculiar attitude of the nation toward the well-being of the race," Du Bois wrote in *The Philadelphia Negro.* There were, he continued, "few other cases in the history of civilized peoples where human suffering has been viewed with such peculiar indifference."

Fifty years after civil rights legislation addressed the legacy of discrimination in housing, education, employment, voting, and other institutions of the country, America remains deeply segregated. Blacks and other people of color are more likely than whites to live in communities with high rates of poverty, where physical and social structures are crumbling, abandoned, and left to die. Even educated, affluent Blacks live in poorer neighborhoods than whites with working-class incomes, which is spelled out in a 2002 report, "Separate and Unequal: The Neighborhood Gap for Blacks and Hispanics in Metropolitan America." Some of this segregation is by choice: many Black people prefer to live in the communities they were raised in, surrounded by a cushion of familiarity, family, and culture. Most of the segregation, though, is not chosen but created by economic forces. Only 44 percent of Black Americans own their homes, compared with about 65 percent of all Americans and 74 percent of whites. Homeownership, a pillar of the so-called American dream, decreased for Black Americans in the decade and a half since 2004, erasing most of the gains made since the passage of the Fair Housing Act in 1968, which outlawed housing discrimination. Numerous studies show that bias by realtors and mortgage lenders contributes to the lack of housing options and opportunities for African Americans. And many Blacks simply cannot afford to buy homes or move. If, like Danielle Bailey-Lash, their property has been devalued by pollution they didn't invite, the problem is compounded. This contributes to a wealth gap between white and Black families that has more than tripled in the last fifty years, according to the Federal Reserve, making the median net worth of white families ten times higher than that of Black families.

Inequality in the conditions of Black communities compared with others is far from new, and racism has been spilled all over the problem for nearly a century. Many areas where the streets remain unsafe, the air and water are dirtiest, and affordable, healthy food and outdoor space are lacking were subject to redlining, a policy that began in the early part of the last century. In the 1930s, the Home Owners' Loan Corporation (HOLC) used color-coded maps that encouraged mortgage lenders to withhold credit from certain communities in 239 cities. These maps graded areas—A ("best"—green), B ("still desirable"—blue), C ("definitely declining"—yellow), and D ("hazardous"—red)—encouraging lending in predominantly white and more affluent areas and discouraging lending in areas with residents of color, especially "Negroes." The Federal Housing Administration later relied on these maps, along with its own underwriting manuals, which resulted in lending institutions issuing fewer mortgages in C and D areas than in other parts of the city, helping to create entrenched segregation, disinvestment, and decay.

Although the practice of redlining was declared illegal in the late 1960s, its impact persists today and has contributed to housing instability, inequitable access to health-promoting resources, and unhealthy living conditions. A 2020 study by the National Community Reinvestment Coalition made an explicit link between the effects of redlining and current health outcomes. Chronic illnesses like asthma, diabetes, hypertension, kidney disease, obesity, and stroke were more prevalent in redlined communities, and life expectancy was cut by 3.6 years in neighborhoods that received the HOLC's D rating.

The Chicago communities where my mother came of age and where residents die young were not just redlined; they were also subject to the predatory practice of contract buying. In the 1950s, speculators created home sale contracts to trap African American families who were eager to purchase homes but whose housing choices were restricted by racial segregation and redlining. These contracts offered Black buyers the false impression of a mortgage but without the protections. Instead, buyers made monthly installments at high interest rates toward bloated purchase prices but did not gain ownership until the contract was paid in full and all conditions met. That meant that contract sellers held the deed of the home and were able to evict the buyers for any missed payments. During the payment period, Black contract buyers accumulated no equity in their homes. According to the 2019 report "The Plunder of Black

Wealth in Chicago," released by the Samuel DuBois Cook Center on Social Equity at Duke University, this practice extracted between $3.2 and $4.0 billion from Chicago's Black community. "The curse of contract sales still reverberates through Chicago's black neighborhoods (and their urban counterparts nationwide)," wrote the Duke researchers, "and helps explain the vast wealth divide between blacks and whites." When I asked my mother how my grandfather managed to scrape together the money to buy the family's first home on East Sixty-Fourth Place sometime in the 1950s, she explained that he didn't have enough for a down payment, so he bought it on contract. "Dad was always terrified about missing a payment because he could lose the building at any time," she told me.

Polluting facilities tend to be located in areas where residents are least able to fight back against them—communities where people of color live and where poor people reside. Stokes County is mostly white. Residents Black and white, middle class and poor, have been exposed to Duke Energy's pollution and poisoned by it since it first located the Belews Creek Steam Station in Walnut Cove the year Danielle and Caroline were born. But the county's poor and Black residents live closest to the plant, the landfills, and the pond and are least able to relocate.

Communities that are both Black and poor have long proven the most vulnerable. Forty years ago, activists began beating the drum about a pattern of situating facilities that contaminate the air, water, and soil—including incinerators, oil refineries, smelters, sewage treatment plants, landfills, and chemical plants—near communities of color, or placing housing where Black, brown, and poor citizens will live close to these kinds of facilities. The first stirrings of the Black-led environmental justice movement date to the late 1970s, out of a convergence of a growing interest in environmental issues with the civil rights and Black Power movements. In 1978, Robert Bullard, then a young professor of sociology at Texas Southern University, walked through the door of his home in Houston and was greeted with the news that his then wife, Linda McKeever Bullard, a lawyer, was suing the City of Houston, Harris County, and the State of Texas—Bullard's employer—in federal court. The suit charged the government agencies, as well as Browning-Ferris Industries, a now-defunct private waste management company, with racial discrimination in siting the Whispering Pines municipal landfill in the predominantly Black Northwood Manor neighborhood in suburban Houston. When they first saw trees being cut down and Bobcats overturning dirt, residents, mostly middle-class homeowners, thought the construction was a shopping mall or new subdivision.

Bullard, who is now a distinguished professor of urban planning and environmental policy at TSU, signed on to help his wife's case.

In the days before internet research, Bullard and a handful of his students combed state and city records on paper or microfiche, walked through neighborhoods using foldout census tract maps, and went door to door, sometimes sticking surveys underneath the wipers of cars in an attempt to locate the waste facilities in the city. Houston is relatively flat, so Bullard advised his students to keep an eye out for hills, which often signaled the site of an old landfill. In the end, they discovered that all five municipal dumps, six of eight city-operated garbage incinerators, and three of four private landfills were located in Black communities—though African Americans made up only 25 percent of the population at that time. Bullard believed the data showed a pattern of biased decisions over years and years by city officials. The siting of Whispering Pines felt like the height of disrespect: the new landfill was thirteen hundred feet from a high school in a Black school district and within two miles of at least half a dozen elementary schools, leaving children smelling garbage in their classrooms on Houston's many hot and humid days.

Though his wife lost the lawsuit and the Whispering Pines landfill still operates, Bullard's work piqued his interest in looking for patterns of environmental racism. In his 1990 book, *Dumping in Dixie: Race, Class, and Environmental Quality*, he argued that pollution from solid waste facilities, hazardous waste landfills, and toxic waste dumps and chemical emissions from industrial facilities were exacting a heavy toll on Black communities across the country. Using case studies—including Sumter County, Alabama, which is the site of the nation's largest hazardous waste landfill—Bullard showed that toxic dumping and unwanted land uses have followed a path of least resistance, meaning they end up sited in Black and poor communities. His book became a bible for the environmental justice movement.

As Bullard was writing *Dumping in Dixie,* residents of Warren County, North Carolina—120 miles north of Walnut Cove—mounted a six-day protest against a toxic landfill being placed in the area of the state with the highest concentration of African Americans and nearly the lowest per capita income. The toxins had an extraordinary origin: In 1978, residents in fourteen North Carolina counties noticed on their way to school, work, and church dark streaks of a greasy substance along the shoulders of 240 miles of roadway. From June to August of that year the Ward Transformer Company sprayed more than thirty thousand gallons of oil thick with polychlorinated biphenyls (PCBs) in the middle of the night, five hundred miles from New York, in order to avoid the cost of proper disposal. The so-called midnight dumpers went to jail, leaving state officials to decide where to place the toxic sludge; PCBs are known to cause birth defects, liver and skin disorders, and cancer. They chose Warren County. In 1982, after several years of organizing, the county made national news when five hundred residents and environmental and civil rights activists were arrested in an effort to stop construction of the Warren County landfill, which was slated to contain sixty thousand tons of contaminated soil. Men, women, and children, both Black and white, held signs that read, "NO PCBs," "We Care About Our Future," and "Dump Hunt in the Dump," referring to North Carolina's then governor, Jim Hunt. A line of Black men, arms behind their heads, lay in the street, blocking dump trucks full of toxic soil, an image that remains an iconic symbol of civil rights activism. A group of mostly women and children, arms locked, clung to each other while being wrenched apart and dragged into buses by state troopers and national guard officers who had been summoned to break up the rallies. The evening news featured dramatic video of prominent Black leaders, watched by highway patrolmen, marching arm in arm with the local organizers as they sang the protest song "Ain't No Stoppin' Us Now."

Though the rallies, marching, arrests, and media attention weren't enough to prevent the landfill from moving forward, they did galvanize a growing environmental justice movement. The following year, the U.S. General Accounting Office examined the link between hazardous waste landfill placement and communities of color. The research found that Blacks made up a majority in three of the four communities with hazardous waste landfills in EPA Region 4, comprising eight southern states. Damning data continued to pile up. In 1987, the United Church of Christ (UCC) Commission for Racial Justice issued a landmark report noting that three out of five Black and Hispanic Americans, or twenty-three million people, resided in communities that housed uncontrolled toxic waste sites, areas where an accumulation of hazardous substances creates a threat to the health and safety of individuals or the environment or both. The study, *Toxic Wastes and Race in the United States,* was the first to examine race, class, and the environment on a national level. It also noted that although socioeconomic status played an important role in the location of hazardous waste sites, race was the most significant factor among the variables analyzed. In 2007, the UCC revisited the research with *Toxic Wastes and Race at Twenty, 1987–2007,* an equally data-driven report with Bullard as a principal author, which found that racial disparities in the location of toxic waste facilities were "greater than previously reported." People of color constituted the majority of the population in communities within 1.8 miles of a polluting facility, and again, race—not income or property values—was the most potent predictor. In time for Black History Month in 2020, the UCC released yet another report, *"Breath to*

the People": Sacred Air and Toxic Pollution, this time partnering
with a nonprofit group called the Environmental Integrity Project.
This new research reinforced what the group first uncovered three
decades earlier: that people of color and the poor are more likely to
live within one mile of the hundred most toxic areas of America.
The authors of this report noted that more than 112,500 children
under age five live within three miles of the nation's one hundred
super-polluting facilities and more than 11,500 live within a mile,
calling the problem "a moral crisis."

Just after the national spotlight shone on Warren County, and the
UCC released its initial report, the federal government was shamed
into action. Early in 1990, the Congressional Black Caucus met
with EPA officials to discuss the poisoning of communities of color
and why the government agency was not addressing the needs of
its constituents. In 1992, the EPA created the Office of Environmental Justice in order to focus on issues of environmental inequality. The new office hired Mustafa Ali, a young Black University of
West Virginia graduate, to serve as an environmental specialist. Born
and raised in West Virginia, in the heart of coal country, Ali had
interned at the EPA through a program designed to recruit people
of color into environmental careers. Once the job offer came, Ali,
then twenty-two, decided to skip a PhD program in Atlanta, cut
his signature hair, which had grown in long waves that grazed the
middle of his back, and work for the federal government. In 1994,
the newly elected president, Bill Clinton, signed into law a bill to
address adverse health and environmental conditions in minority
and low-income populations. The government also established a
multimillion-dollar grants program to support grassroots organizations working on environmental justice issues.

The changes at the EPA dovetailed neatly with the environmental
justice movement happening on the ground. Ali had a foot in both
worlds. At the time, there were still people in senior positions in the
Environmental Protection Agency and other places who believed
that the impacts on these communities weren't real and that local

residents had to be imagining or exaggerating the pollution and its effects. Over the next two decades and under four presidents, Ali would climb the ranks until, in 2008, he was named director of the Office of Environmental Justice and special adviser to the EPA administrator on environmental justice issues. Though during his tenure the EPA was criticized for not doing enough to combat environmental issues in communities of color and poor communities and the Flint water catastrophe also unfolded during his term, Ali and his colleagues assisted fifteen hundred communities with small grants to address local environmental issues.

Then, in 2017, Donald Trump appointed Scott Pruitt to head the EPA. Before he could decorate his D.C. office, Pruitt, a climate change denier and friend of the fossil fuel industry who as Oklahoma's attorney general sued the EPA multiple times, proposed to gut the agency's budget from $8 to $6 billion and reduce the agency's staff of fifteen thousand by 20 percent. The proposal also called for dismantling the Office of Environmental Justice and eliminating the small grants program, and Ali soon noticed that the new cast of EPA administrators had begun to ice him out of meetings. In March 2017, after calling his parents, talking to his mentors, and praying, Ali made the gut-wrenching decision to resign from the EPA. On March 8, 2017, he turned in his resignation, just short of twenty-five years at the agency, which meant he would not qualify for his full pension. But he didn't go out quietly. His three-page, single-spaced resignation letter to Pruitt detailed the agency's environmental justice successes and pleaded with eloquence and urgency but not bitterness that the EPA not turn its back on marginalized communities. "Administrator Pruitt, you have a once-in-a-lifetime opportunity to bring people together," he wrote, "to ensure that all communities have safe places to live, learn, work, play and pray and to ensure that our most vulnerable communities, who have been struggling for clean air to breathe and clean water to drink becomes a reality for them and their children." The letter went viral and has reportedly been viewed more than one million times. Before his last day on the job, Ali says he tried to meet with Pruitt, to look his boss in the eye and share his viewpoint respectfully, but the EPA administrator refused. Ali went on to become vice president for environmental justice, climate, and community revitalization at the National Wildlife Federation, and his EPA position was never filled. A year and a half later, in July 2018, Scott Pruitt resigned in the face of a dozen ethics investigations, including lavish spending for foreign travel and purchasing a $43,000 secure phone booth with taxpayer funds. Before Pruitt was pushed out, an arm of his agency, the National Center for Environmental Assessment, released a report that showed that Black Americans are exposed to 1.5 times more air pollutants that contribute to issues like heart and lung disease than white people, and people living in poverty had 1.3 times the exposure of those who are not poor. Pruitt was replaced by Andrew Wheeler, also a climate change denier, who spent much of his career as a lobbyist for the coal industry.

Danielle took a tentative step into the environmental justice spotlight in 2018. The previous year, the Reverend Dr. William Barber, the civil rights activist and MacArthur genius, had resurrected the Poor People's Campaign. Reverend Barber's twenty-first-century version of the Reverend Dr. Martin Luther King Jr.'s war on poverty pointed to ecological destruction and climate change as pillars of the campaign. The campaign outline states, "Our policies have not fundamentally valued human life or the ecological systems in which we live. Instead, it has prioritized private, corporate and financial interests over our precious natural resources . . . We have a fundamental right to clean water, air and a healthy environment and public resources to monitor, penalize and reverse the polluting impacts of fossil fuel industries."

Along with the former vice president Al Gore, Barber took a two-day swing through North Carolina, where Barber was raised and has spent much of his life, in order to see the effects of environmental racism for himself and talk directly to people living in polluted communities. At the same time the campaign was examining pollution in North Carolina's poor communities and communities of color,

Donald Trump's EPA overhauled Obama administration regulations on coal ash, giving industry and states more authority over its disposal. The week after the North Carolina tour, the EPA would relax rules on air pollution from coal-fired plants like the Belews Creek Steam Station, even as the agency predicted the change would cause up to fourteen hundred deaths a year over the next decade.

On August 13, Reverend Barber and Gore joined a roomful of Walnut Cove residents—as well as local and national media—in the chapel of the Rising Star Baptist Church. On that day, which was her forty-fifth birthday, Danielle nervously approached the lectern, her hair falling in a thick sheet over the surgical scar on the right side of her head. It was her first time speaking in public on a national stage. "I used to live on Pine Hall Road about three miles from Belews Creek," she began, her voice unsteady. "I thought it was such a blessing to have that house, because we could walk down our driveway through the woods and get in the water. We would swim in that water, eat the fish from the water. How did I not know it was dangerous to live near a power plant?"

As she continued the story of her symptoms and brain cancer diagnosis, she mentioned Caroline, and the importance of their friendship, and Caroline moved from another part of the room to stand by her friend's side. "I believe that God kept me alive for a purpose," said Danielle. "I never knew what my purpose was, but now I know my purpose is to fight this good fight. The same way that I had to believe that I was healed when they told me I was going to die is the same faith that I have to believe that we are going to win this fight."

Later, Reverend Barber held a press conference on the boat ramp of Belews Lake's Pine Hall Road entrance, the lake looking murky and green in the background. Leaning heavily on a cane, Reverend Barber, a mountain of a man, spoke to the crowd in his blistering baritone. He shared a story of challenging an elected official who had suggested coal ash wasn't a real problem. "If the coal ash is not that problematic, then you go down, get some coal ash in a jar and drink some of that coal ash," he told *The Stokes News.* "Don't tell us that it's alright. I bet you they don't have coal ash dumping around the governor's mansion. I bet you your legislature isn't anywhere near a coal ash pond. I bet you don't find it in wealthy communities."

Danielle's heartfelt testimony in her hometown struck a chord with Gore and his daughter Karenna, the director of Earth Ethics at Union Theological Seminary, and she was invited to the main stage at the Climate Reality Project's Leadership Corps Training in Atlanta in mid-March 2019. The brainchild of Al Gore, this event attracted two thousand mostly young white activists who had come to learn about environmental and climate justice. Despite the project's efforts to reflect the communities most affected by environmental poisoning, Reverend Barber, Robert Bullard, Mustafa Ali, and a handful of others were the rare Black faces in a sea of white activists. At this point, after a third craniotomy, Danielle was using a wearable device called Optune to keep the cancer at bay. Created specifically for patients with glioblastoma, it produces low-intensity, wavelike electric fields through adhesive patches attached to the skull to slow or stop cancer cells from dividing, and at best to destroy them. The device runs continuously, powered by a portable charger. Caroline accompanied Danielle from Walnut Cove to Atlanta to help her get through airport security with the Optune and handle the bulky medical equipment.

On Thursday, March 14, at 11:00 a.m., Danielle took the stage to speak on a panel called "Stories from the Frontlines: The Climate Crisis, a Social Justice Crisis." She joined Russel Honoré, a retired lieutenant general who coordinated the military relief efforts for Hurricane Katrina; the Reverend Paul Wilson, pastor of Union Hill and Union Grove Baptist Churches, in Union Hill, Virginia, a town founded by enslaved Black people that was in a bare-knuckle battle against Dominion Energy, which planned to locate a gas-fire compressor station that would release toxic emissions into the area; and Katherine Cummings, an activist who fought against the siting of a coal-burning power plant eight miles from her home in rural

Georgia. The discussion was moderated by Gore in a cavernous room in the Georgia World Congress Center. Danielle, wearing a light-brown turban with knit flowers on the right side as well as her battery backpack, looked small and tentative, sandwiched onstage between two of the men, her hands folded in her lap. In the program she was described only as an "impacted community member." But as she spoke, the audience quieted. In her natural self-effacing way, she said she felt "stupid" for swimming in Belews Lake and eating fish from it, and shifted attention to Caroline, who was watching her from the audience, crediting her friend with urging her to move away from the plant. Though she spoke the least onstage, dwarfed by several big personalities, including Gore's, when Danielle described surviving past her three- to six-month expiration date, threw up her hands, smiled, and said, "But here I am," the audience applauded. Two weeks after the conference in Atlanta, the activism of Danielle and her scrappy neighbors would pay off: on April 1, the North Carolina Department of Environmental Quality ordered Duke Energy to remove all coal ash from nine basins at six plants in the state, including the Belews Creek station. The good news was short-lived: almost immediately, Duke announced it would fight the order, returning to court to insist that rather than dig up the toxic ash and move it away from where people live, it would keep it in place in those locations, sealed with a cap.

Though Black people like Danielle bear the physical and emotional hardships of the environmental crisis, they tend to be left out of the membership and leadership of the environmental movement. That means that though some notable Black environmental activists have broken through—including Bullard, Ali, Beverly Wright, Catherine Flowers, Will Allen, Majora Carter, and Peggy Shepard—the face of environmental activism is more likely to be Greta Thunberg, the spunky Swedish teenager who was named *Time* magazine's 2019 Person of the Year, not someone like Danielle living environmental injustice on the ground. Protests and movement conferences like Gore's are filled with mostly young white people, not Black people whose families have lived near polluting facilities for generations, their bodies ravaged by the effects of toxic emissions.

The homogeneity of the mainstream environmental establishment spurred the emergence of a Black-led environmental justice movement. In 1990, with the media spotlight on the protests in Warren County, North Carolina, and the evidence from the United Church of Christ study proving that African Americans suffer most from pollution, activists on the ground got little support from organizations like Greenpeace, the National Audubon Society, the National Wildlife Federation, the National Resources Defense Council, the Nature Conservancy, the Sierra Club, and the World Wildlife Fund. In March 1990, more than a hundred grassroots activists signed a letter accusing the ten most prominent environmental groups of racism. The letter pointed to the lack of people of color in decision-making roles and to inaction in addressing the environmental problems of oppressed communities. In the end, the activists demanded that this group of ten cease operations in communities of color within sixty days until they had increased staffing of people of color to between 35 and 40 percent. That didn't happen. The following year, more than five hundred people gathered in Washington, D.C., for the First National People of Color Environmental Leadership Summit. The weekend event in 1991 produced a seventeen-point platform to combat environmental racism and also helped dispel the assumption that Black and brown people are not interested in or active on environmental issues. The first point: "Environmental justice affirms the sacredness of Mother Earth, ecological unity and the interdependence of all species, and the right to be free from ecological destruction."

Over the years, the broader movement has nodded toward diversity. Bullard, one of the organizers of the 1991 conference, who has written or co-authored eighteen books about environmental justice and is widely known as the father of environmental justice, founded the HBCU Climate Change Consortium in 2011 with a colleague, Beverly Wright. Their goal is to diversify the leadership of the environmental movement. A 2018 survey conducted by Yale University professor Dorceta Taylor found that white people made up 85 percent of the staffs and 80 percent of the boards of 2,057 environmental nonprofits despite making up 60 percent of the population. A 2019 report released by Green 2.0, a working group that examines the intersection of the environment and race, showed that people of color make up only 4 percent of the senior staff of 40 environmental foundations.

By the fall of 2019, the order to force Duke to clean up the coal ash mess remained tied up in court, and Danielle's health had begun to decline. When shaving her head to accommodate the Optune device, her mother found a worrisome bump on her daughter's skull. Danielle was also losing weight and had become alarmingly thin—shrinking from a size 12 to a 4. Still, she remained positive and urged everyone around her to do the same, and she pushed her life forward. She resumed taking classes at Guilford Technical Community College in Greensboro and continued to be active in both her church and the environmental groups fighting to get Duke to do the right thing. The activism and public spotlight had ignited something in Danielle, and she decided to run for a seat on the Town of Walnut Cove Board of Commissioners.

At the end of October, a biopsy of the bump her mother had uncovered showed that the cancer had come roaring back. By then, both her mom and Caroline also noticed cognitive changes. Danielle would sometimes become disoriented, lose her purse, forget how to get home from a trip to the store, or not recognize people she had known for years, including her children. On November 5, she won the election, but rather than be excited, she seemed confused. When Caroline gave her friend a congratulatory hug, she seemed not to recognize her. A few days after her victory, Danielle was admitted to the hospital, and her condition worsened until eventually she transitioned to hospice care. She passed away just before midnight on November 30, her sister Michelle at her bedside. Danielle was forty-five years old.

On December 31, 2019, the residents of Walnut Cove finally and definitively won the fight against Duke Energy. The company reached a settlement with the state Department of Environmental Quality and agreed to remove eighty million tons of coal ash from around the state. The substance would be excavated and placed in lined storage pits to avoid leakage that further poisons the soil and water. Caroline and about forty local activists and members of Appalachian Voices gathered on Saturday, January 18, 2020, to celebrate the victory. But it felt bittersweet: they had won the battle but lost Danielle, whose memory hung over the event, whose absence stung.

Still, Danielle's legacy and the positive spirit she insisted on linger. Her mother, Sandra, visits her daughter's grave site on sunny days. Danielle is buried on the edge of Fairview Cemetery in London, one of three Black communities in the area. When I traveled to Stokes County in 2020, the site was designated with a simple metal marker, while the family decided on a proper gravestone. Danielle's mom had wedged a bright bouquet of pink silk roses on top. She prefers them to real flowers, which wilt and die and make her feel sad. At home, she keeps the nameplate of the office her daughter was never able to fill: Danielle Bailey-Lash, Commissioner. She was the first Black woman elected to the board of commissioners of their town and would've been the first to serve. The gold nameplate sits in the front of a bookshelf, behind a collage of photographs of Danielle. On February 21, about three months after his mother's death, Danielle's son, Anthony, and his wife had their second child. They named her Eyden Danielle.

Caroline thinks about her friend every day, sometimes several times, and is determined to keep her memory alive. In 2018, inspired by Danielle, she created the Lilies Project, a grant-funded initiative, with the goal of making public art out of coal ash. In early 2020, Caroline unveiled the first of three labyrinths made of bricks manufactured at a facility not far from Danielle's home that contain trace amounts of coal ash. That first installment, inlaid in a grassy yard behind Christ Episcopal Church near the center of town, will be followed by a concrete labyrinth in a public park and a third made of canvas to be used at various community groups. All of this art will be part of a guided tour of the town. Caroline chose the labyrinth, a twisty maze, with one single circuitous path to the center and out again, as a symbol of all Danielle stood for: spirituality, beauty, courage, healing, dignity, and love.

CHAPTER SIX

STRONG, LOUD, AND ANGRY: THE INVISIBILITY OF BLACK EMOTIONAL PAIN

On a hectic day in April 2019, the Hollywood stylist Audrey Brianne took a belt out of her closet, put it around her neck, and decided to end her life. The death of her younger brother Jason in 2015 from diabetes, along with the murder of one of her closest friends by a stalker the following year, sent Brianne into an emotional downward spiral. One of the few Black stylists consistently dressing celebrities for awards shows and red-carpet events, she felt extreme pressure to perform, giving her no time to catch her breath or grieve her loved ones. Buoyed by vodka, which she bought by the handle and consumed from 7:00 a.m., when she got up, until 2:00 a.m., when her head hit the pillow, she pushed herself through seven-day workweeks, keeping up the grind, afraid to say no. She worked hard but appeared easygoing and accommodating, in an attempt to battle back stereotypes of Black women as loud, angry, and trifling. She was always available to her clients, phone number never on do not disturb, until the weight of the job, the deaths, and the depression that had been dragging her down, off and on, since high school finally pulled her under. Still, as she stood in her condo in Los Angeles, depressed and depleted, she realized she didn't actually want to die, but she also didn't know how to live with the bottomless pain and darkness that had seeped into every corner of her life. So instead of hanging herself, she turned to her phone and googled "suicide hotline." When a calm voice answered the 800 call, she told him, "I'm having a really hard time right now, and I almost just did something really stupid." He stayed on the line with her for two hours and brought her back from the brink.

Black Americans have long lived under tremendous emotional pressure in the face of bias and inequality, much of it sanctioned by the government and embedded in the structures and institutions of society since the earliest days of the country. Just as high-effort coping eats away at the physical health of Black Americans—as framed by Arline Geronimus and her theory of weathering on the body—struggling against discrimination frays and fractures their mental health. A 2018 national survey by the Substance Abuse and Mental Health Services Administration found that African Americans are 20 percent more likely to have serious psychological distress than whites; they are also more likely than whites to report persistent symptoms such as sadness, hopelessness, and feeling as if everything seems like a struggle. Poverty worsens this struggle, but even people like Audrey Brianne, who have achieved success in their industries, get worn down emotionally by the macro- and microaggressions, slights, and subtle, often indirect, forms of discrimination they face when working, learning, and living in predominantly white spaces. This can result in everything from fatigue to feelings of failure and anger and can trigger depression or other forms of mental illness. For those who are already suffering from mental health issues, it can become dangerous and life threatening. The proliferation of high-profile police killings of Black people in recent years has created repeated trauma and stress; a 2018 study at the University of Pennsylvania's Perelman School of Medicine found that police killings of unarmed African Americans have adverse effects on mental health among Black American adults who were not directly affected by the incident.

Understanding and confronting mental illness remain difficult for nearly everyone, regardless of race. A lack of sympathy for the mentally ill—and a dearth of understanding of mental illness—exacerbate this problem in the United States, where public stigma motivates people to fear, reject, and discriminate against those with mental illness. Despite public information campaigns costing tens of millions of dollars, Americans are suspicious of people with severe mental illness, believing them to always be violent. In fact, the vast majority aren't. Instead, they are much more likely to be victimized by violence than the general population. Deinstitutionalization has driven significant numbers of mentally ill people into public spaces, where they are vulnerable. This government policy, which dates to the 1960s, led to a decline in treatment options for those suffering from serious psychiatric disorders. A 2012 report by the Treatment Advocacy Center found the number of inpatient treatment beds in state psychiatric facilities decreased further by 14 percent from 2005 to 2010, leaving only 14 available beds per 100,000 people. Instead, those who could have been living in a psychiatric facility or treated at a hospital—men and women with schizophrenia, severe bipolar disorder, and other mental illnesses—are far too often living in or spending the bulk of their days in public places such as libraries, parks, and mass transit, without affordable access to comprehensive treatment. If they become disruptive, there is a good chance someone will call the police.

For Black people struggling with mental illness, the perception that they are violent is compounded by racist stereotypes, creating extreme intolerance, a lack of empathy, and fear. In fact, even as they may be viewed as violent, and punished for it, far too many Black Americans suffer mental illness in silence because of the false idea that emotional struggles signal weakness. They may also believe suffering is their lot. In Zora Neale Hurston's 1937 novel, *Their Eyes Were Watching God,* Janie's grandmother tells her, "De nigger woman is de mule uh de world so fur as Ah can see." Black women, she is saying, faced with both racism and sexism, bear the weight of the world, without praise or even thanks. That kind of belief explains why emotional pain can go unnoticed by individuals even as they suffer, under the assumption that it is an inextricable part of the Black experience in America, a burden to be endured or ignored.

Audrey Brianne's dance with her demons began at age fifteen. Her father, a telecommunications executive, started a new job and relocated his wife and four children from Denver to Palo Alto in 1999. In that city in Northern California, Blacks make up about 2 percent of the population. To fit in at her new school, Audrey joined the swim team. With her brown skin and thick body constantly on display in practice and at meets, Audrey felt depressed and out of place, and by age sixteen she had developed an eating disorder. Bulimia led to rapid weight loss, but she flew under the radar: it has long been incorrectly assumed by mental health providers as well as in the Black community that Black women don't suffer from eating disorders. Bulimia and anorexia have historically been associated with young, white women, though in reality they affect people from all demographics of all ethnicities at similar rates. A 2009 study found that Black teens are 50 percent more likely to binge and purge yet receive treatment much less frequently. A 2020 review of thirty-eight previous studies again corrected the false assumption that Black women are immune to eating disorders and added that research on eating disorders has focused on white women, with Black people underrepresented in clinical trials.

At first, Audrey received praise for losing weight. But as she got smaller and smaller—she eventually lost more than sixty pounds, her clothing size reduced to a 0—her parents grew alarmed. And it wasn't just the weight loss that frightened Audrey's parents; they could see that their daughter was not herself. Audrey describes her sadness as a kind of heaviness that she had to carry. Her parents forced her into therapy, but Audrey was sullen and uncooperative during her sessions. She would sit in the therapist's office for an hour, silent and defiant. Eventually, she switched to group therapy, focused on teens with eating issues; she was the only Black person in the group. Even at her lowest point emotionally, she maintained an A average and stayed on the honor roll. During her senior year, the family relocated back to Denver and settled in Cherry Creek, a section where Blacks make up a tiny proportion of the population.

Audrey was better now; she had put some of the weight back on and had discovered a love of fashion through a club at her high school. In 2002, she enrolled in the University of Colorado at Boulder, a large public university with more than thirty-six thousand students, only about 2 percent of them Black, and pledged Gamma Phi Beta, an almost all-white sorority. Though her mental health and weight were more stable in college, she remembers finding it difficult and lonely to constantly "integrate" the classrooms she studied in, the dorms she lived in, and later the fashion internships and early jobs in Los Angeles, where she landed after college.

When I met Audrey, I empathized with her about the often silent toll it takes to constantly be an "only"; living with mental illness makes it even more challenging for her. I also grew up in Denver and went to the University of Colorado. In fact, I introduced myself to her at a CU alumni event in 2021 where she discussed her struggles with emotional health. As she shared her story that day, I thought about the long-standing perception that suicide is a white problem; Black people die from homicide, whites from suicide, the assumption goes, despite research that points to a concerning increase in suicidal behavior among Black youth since the early 1990s. I was also keenly reminded of another successful Black woman who drove herself to impossibly high standards while grappling with crippling depression: Leanita McClain, who gained fame three decades earlier as a face of tragedy.

By all measures, McClain, a journalist, had achieved success. In 1984, she was a columnist for the *Chicago Tribune* and the first Black and second woman to join the publication's powerful editorial board. Her twice-weekly column reached one million readers. McClain had first gained national prominence four years earlier at the age of twenty-nine when she published an essay about race called "The Middle-Class Black's Burden" in *Newsweek*. In it, she described the strain of having a foot in two worlds: the housing project on the South Side of Chicago where she had been raised and the nearly all-white upper echelons of journalism where she had landed. The double bind she felt surfaced early in a poem she wrote in high school. It begins, "I should like to die in winter / When my blood upon the snow / Will leave a clue to those who pass / Of my brief, futile life," and ends, "And none will learn the truth of the matter. / My secret will melt with the snow. / But the spot will run red each winter hence. / Though I be rotted below." And though having a My Turn column in *Newsweek* is a high point in any career, McClain's also reads like a cry for help. "I have a foot in each world, but I cannot fool myself about either," she wrote. "I can see the transparent deceptions of some whites and the bitter hopelessness of some blacks. I know how tenuous my grip on one way of life is, and how strangling the grip of the other way of life can be."

Hiding behind a meticulously maintained outward-facing image, McClain was struggling with serious depression. After a suicide attempt in 1981, she was hospitalized and prescribed psychiatric medication by her physician. On May 29, 1984, she swallowed a handful of antidepressants that she had stockpiled and died alone. In one of six suicide notes she left behind, she wrote, "Happiness is a private club that will not let me enter. As my dreams will never come true, I choose to have them in perpetual sleep." Her suicide sent shock waves through journalism circles across the country. Her early poetry, journalistic work, and suicide notes were compiled in a posthumous book, *A Foot in Each World*, edited by her former husband, the journalist Clarence Page.

The public relations executive Terrie Williams sent similar shocks through the Black community in 2005 with a personal essay published in *Essence* titled "Depression and the Superwoman." Williams too had "made it." Trained as a social worker, she switched gears in 1988 and opened the Terrie Williams Agency, a PR firm with Miles Davis and Eddie Murphy as early clients. By the time I met her sometime in the 1990s, she was widely considered *the* publicist to Black Hollywood and over the years represented Prince, Janet Jackson, Al Sharpton, Johnnie Cochran, and many other luminaries. But in 2003, Williams experienced a soul-crushing bout of depression. It had been sneaking up on her, but she ignored the signs, keeping on her game face while, like Audrey Brianne, running herself ragged in service of her business and clients' needs. Eventually, the pain built to an unbearable degree and she collapsed, unable to get out of bed for days. In 2005, *Essence*'s editor in chief, Susan L. Taylor, persuaded her to share her story, including the shame she felt as she coped with the taboo of mental illness among Black Americans and her path to healing. There is no way to describe the collective relief thousands of Black women felt when Williams explained how depression forced her to pull off the mask, take off the Superwoman cape, and stop hiding, lying, and pretending she was okay. She received ten thousand letters and followed up in 2008 with a very popular book, *Black Pain: It Just Looks Like We're Not Hurting*. The title still strikes a chord.

Millions of African Americans struggle with mental illness, yet only 33 percent of them receive mental health treatment each year, compared with the U.S. average of 44 percent of all those who suffer. Research shows that African Americans are more likely to turn to emergency rooms or primary care physicians during a mental health crisis, or receive no help for emotional distress at all. Why don't the majority of Black people with mental health challenges get needed care? First, stigma. Instead of seeking psychological help—or sometimes help of any kind, even from loved ones—Black women especially choose to carry the load, often turning to religion when facing mental health issues, most commonly depression. Living in communities that lack adequate transportation and health-care facilities creates additional hurdles to getting affordable treatment for mental illness or help at all. A history of distrust in the medical system includes lack of confidence in mental health providers; Black Americans often don't trust that health-care professionals of all kinds have their best interests at heart. If they are dealing with additional personal issues, such as sexuality or gender identity, it can compound feelings of isolation and create fear of seeking help.

For those who overcome the stigma and look for help, getting good treatment for mental illness can be challenging. The vast majority of mental health treatment providers in the United States are white: about 84 percent of the psychology workforce is white and 4 percent Black, according to American Psychological Association data. Even the most well-meaning white mental health providers may lack the cultural competence to deal with patients whose experience doesn't match theirs.

Black patients understand this. Stories are rampant, both in academic studies and in everyday life, of misdiagnosis and under-treatment for Black people experiencing mental health issues. This includes Black people who are struggling with severe depression being misdiagnosed as schizophrenic and Black mothers, who are at a greater risk for postpartum depression, being less likely to receive care. Problems with diagnosis or treatment are fueled by persistent stereotypes of Black people as angry, dangerous, overly emotional, and impervious to pain, or, paradoxically, so strong and resourceful that they don't need help.

Mistreatment of African Americans in the mental health field dates back centuries. During the transatlantic slave trade, Black men were described as having "primitive psychological organization" that made them "uniquely fitted for bondage," according to the authors Alexander Thomas and Samuel Sillen in their 1972 book, *Racism and Psychiatry*. One of the signers of the Declaration of Independence, Benjamin Rush, known as the father of American psychiatry, believed that Black people suffered from a medical affliction called Negritude, which he described as a "disorder" akin to a mild form of leprosy. With his insistence that enslaved Blacks suffered from drapetomania—a mental illness that caused them to attempt escape—Dr. Samuel Cartwright of New Orleans may be added to the list of physicians and medical "experts" who used science to claim that Black people were mentally deficient.

Fast-forward a century: in the 1960s, during the civil rights movement and at a time of increased Black leadership in political, academic, and corporate spaces, the scientific community began to describe schizophrenia as a violent social disease that afflicted Negro men. A 1968 article in the publication *Archives of General Psychia-*

try described schizophrenia as a "protest psychosis" in which Black men developed "hostile and aggressive feelings." As schizophrenia came to be seen as synonymous with antisocial, violent Black men, the association was used as justification for laws that treated mental illness as a criminal, not medical, condition. Rehabilitation was swapped out for efforts to control Black men through law enforcement. Black men are still four times more likely than white men to be diagnosed with schizophrenia, according to an often-cited 2019 Rutgers University study; the researchers concluded that clinicians put more emphasis on psychotic than on depressive symptoms in African Americans, leading to an overuse of diagnoses of schizophrenia. Consequently, Black men are also underdiagnosed with posttraumatic stress and mood disorders.

Untreated mental illness can make African Americans more vulnerable to substance abuse, homelessness, suicide, and homicide. And this begins with Black youth. Between 1991 and 2017, suicide attempts decreased among teens in every ethnic group except for African Americans. Instead, according to a 2019 study published in the journal *Pediatrics,* suicide attempts among Black children and teenagers increased by 73 percent. Among Black boys specifically, attempts climbed 122 percent during the same time period.

Over the years, as she grappled with mental health issues, Audrey Brianne felt an overwhelming sense of shame, which she kept tucked away. It took her years to ask for help because she felt that if she did, she couldn't maintain the image of the strong Black woman who was resilient against anything. If she succumbed to the depression, she believed, she was letting down the Black community. She also feared she'd lose the business she started in 2011 if her clients knew she was so depressed. Her tenuous place in predominantly white Hollywood magnified the anxiety. But eventually, overwhelmed and afraid, she asked for support. In 2018, after she hung up with the National Suicide Prevention Lifeline, she picked up the phone and called her mother and told her, "Mommy, I need help."

With her parents' assistance, she found an inpatient facility in Arizona where she was treated for secondary PTSD as a result of the murder of her friend and substance abuse. She told her clients she was taking a "hiatus." At the facility, where she remained for forty-five days, she was the only Black person in a population of more than two hundred patients. She understands that most people, especially most Black people, can't afford the treatment her parents paid for—roughly the equivalent of a four-year college education. "It's not fair," she says. "There's this whole other group and community that have the same kind of struggles and hurts that isn't even being represented in the room. Mental health care should be free."

After rehab, when Audrey returned to Los Angeles, she didn't trust herself to avoid drinking and moved into a sober-living house, which prohibited substance use of any kind, monitoring patients with urine samples and Breathalyzer tests. She then moved back into her own home, but continued outpatient treatment that involved daily group and individual therapy. When I spoke to her in 2021, she was stable with the help of psychiatric medication, had returned to work, and hadn't touched alcohol in two years.

Black men are even less likely to recognize mental illness and seek treatment; the intersection of race and masculinity puts pressure on them to conform to traditional gender norms of toughness, fearlessness, and invulnerability to pain. And in both Black men and Black women, but men especially, the crossroads where race, uncontrolled mental illness, and law enforcement meet has become particularly dangerous. The story of Mark McMullen offers a tragic illustration.

Over Labor Day weekend in 2011, it seemed as though Mark's life was finally headed in the right direction. He had recently married and was an attentive father to his young son, Simon. A talented chef who had discovered a passion for cooking as a boy, Mark had spent two years at the Cordon Bleu Culinary Institute in Chicago and had amassed extensive experience working in professional kitchens across the country. In 1993, he even helped prepare a gala dinner for Julia Child in honor of her eightieth birthday that was covered by *The New York Times* and aired on PBS. In early September 2011,

Mark's mother, Gloria, had organized a family gathering in part to honor her youngest son and to show support for and celebrate his new life. After a trip to Lake Compounce amusement park in Bristol, Connecticut, Mark and his parents, wife, son, sister, niece, and two uncles returned to the McMullen family home in Middletown, Connecticut, to continue the festivities. Sitting at the kitchen table where decades ago he had served meals to his older siblings after school by throwing together whatever was in the fridge, he excitedly shared plans for the Copper Lobster. He hoped to open this restaurant on Martha's Vineyard, where he had spent time during the summers of his childhood and later as an adult. Best of all, he promised—swore—that after seven stints at rehab centers, and several periods of incarceration for misconduct related to addiction, his battle with drugs, which he used to ease the terror associated with bipolar disorder, had finally ended. His mother, his ride or die in his more than two-decade battle with mental illness and addiction, finally allowed herself a sliver of hope.

But the restaurant never happened, and his family never got the chance to say goodbye. Mark's wife, Kety, would never see him alive again, and their son was destined to grow up not knowing his father. Beginning Tuesday evening September 6, Mark's drug use, complicated by mental illness, came hurtling back and intersected tragically with Boston police officers operating outside their jurisdiction. On Wednesday, September 7, Mark McMullen was shot to death surrounded by a wall of police vehicles. While Mark, unarmed, was sitting inside his father's car, the Boston PD officer Christopher Carr opened fire at point-blank range, striking him in the arms and chest. Carr and another officer were subsequently cleared of all charges, and Carr was later rewarded for murdering Mark.

How did Mark McMullen, the forty-four-year-old son of a university professor, from a close-knit African American family of strivers, who was more sick than dangerous, end up in a fatal altercation with police and become a statistic in a death scroll of African Americans murdered by the police?

The fundamental answer is that behavior caused by mental illness is far too often treated as a crime. Forty percent of adults with serious mental illnesses will come into contact with the criminal justice system during their lives, according to the National Alliance on Mental Illness. Individuals with severe mental illnesses generate no less than one in ten calls for police service and occupy at least one in five of America's prison and jail beds. Jails and prisons hold more people with serious mental illnesses—several hundred thousand individuals—than hospitals. Most are charged with minor misdemeanor crimes and low-level felonies directly tied to their psychiatric illnesses.

Yet once in police custody, the outcome for a Black suspect with mental illness is too often dire. By all accounts, including databases of fatal police encounters kept by *The Washington Post* and *The Guardian,* one in four fatal encounters ends the life of an individual with severe mental illness. At this rate, the risk of being killed during a police encounter is sixteen times greater for individuals with untreated mental illness than for other civilians approached or stopped by officers.

Add to this that Black people in general are more likely than others to be killed by police during encounters with law enforcement, its own public health crisis. According to Mapping Police Violence, a website that tracks information on police violence and use of force, Black people are 3 times more likely to be killed by the police compared with whites and 1.3 times more likely to be unarmed when they are. The deadly through line of all these statistics is that the mentally ill person pulled into the criminal justice system and harmed or killed by law enforcement is disproportionately likely to be Black and most commonly is a Black man.

Mark McMullen was born in Boston, the youngest of Ronald and Gloria McMullen's three children. Allen, Ronald's son from an earlier relationship, sometimes stayed with the family. In 1970, the McMullens moved to Middletown, where Ronald, a lifelong educator en route to a doctorate in applied behavioral science, was hired as assistant director of Wesleyan University's Upward Bound program, which offered college readiness support for first-generation students and those from racial, ethnic, and economic groups underrepresented in higher education. The family eventually settled in a two-story, three-bedroom colonial house on East Street in a pastoral area of Middletown. The suburban community was about 80 percent white at the time, in sharp contrast to Roxbury, where the children had been born, and Mattapan, where the family had moved from. The racial fit was sometimes uncomfortable for the family.

The adjustment was easiest for Mark, who was a toddler when the McMullens relocated. By the time he started kindergarten, it was clear that Mark's upbeat personality and creative spirit would serve him well for bridging the racial divide. He made friends easily. Mark's older siblings, who remember sometimes feeling lonely, isolated, and unwelcome in Middletown, both marveled and made fun of the ragtag crew of friends their baby brother collected and played with. They called his boys the FOACs—"fresh out of the cradle," since most were younger than Mark. Outgoing, personable, energetic, and engaged, he liked to swim, ski, bowl, and draw. Mark loved animals, including the assortment of McMullen family pets, a cat, a gerbil, goldfish, turtles, and a dog named Augie. In later life, he gave up eating meat because he cared about animals so much. Mark was a Cub Scout, and one year the car he made won the Pinewood Derby.

Cooking, however, was Mark's passion, even as a young child. In early 1978, Gloria McMullen returned to work after years of raising her children and taking care of the home. That meant that when the bus dropped off Chris and Karen from high school, and Mark from middle school, they waited for their parents to get home, often hungry for a snack. All of the McMullens tell the same story about Mark: While his older siblings would open the refrigerator, look inside, and complain that there was nothing to eat, when Mark looked in the fridge, he saw possibility. "We would hear him in the kitchen banging around and he'd come in with spaghetti and meatballs, garlic bread," recalls Karen McMullen, laughing. "We're like, 'Where'd you get that?' He's like, 'I made it. Want some?'"

During middle school, though, Mark's wild energy became too large for the small town, and he began to get into trouble. It started with low-level misconduct—shooting at parked cars with a BB gun and being disruptive in school. His parents switched him from Keigwin Middle School to a private school that eventually asked him to leave. In 1982, on his sister's high school graduation day, Mark took his mother's car and wrecked it. His parents became increasingly alarmed by their youngest son's behavior and also worried about his drawings. His sketches were well executed, his talent apparent, but they were frightening. His mother describes the artwork as "dark"—pencil drawings of muscular warriors, their faces demonic and contorted in rage. In a yellowed sketch pad, Mark had drawn a series of angry figures, one robotic, another a severed torso; at the top of the page he wrote, "I killed them, yes, I killed all of them."

Mark's distressed parents took their fifteen-year-old son to a therapist in the area in 1982. Ronald McMullen, with his background in psychology, was particularly insistent that they get their son psychological testing. Gloria can't recall what the therapist told them about Mark, but it wasn't helpful. Years later, as an adult and in the throes of drug addiction, Mark visited another mental health professional, who diagnosed him with bipolar disorder. But he was never given consistent treatment. Gloria rummages through boxes and boxes of files she's amassed documenting the decades she spent trying to understand what was going on with her youngest son and trying to help him. But she can't find among the medical records that scrap of paper that confirmed Mark's bipolar diagnosis.

Looking at the past backward through the clear-eyed lens of history, the signs were all there. His manic, "up" phases were most obvious. At the time, though, his family believed that Mark's emotional intensity, seductive charm, feelings of invincibility, impulsivity, risk taking, nonstop ideas—many unrealized—bursts of creative activity, and boundless talking were just part of who he was. One of the boxes in the McMullen attic is stuffed with notebooks full of menus for restaurants Mark dreamed of starting. There are lists of recipes, in his scratchy handwriting, that he hoped to prepare and serve. One spiral binder contains several dozen dishes listed at the top of blank pages—Bacon Leek Quiche, Roast Beet Salad, Sweet Pea Beurre Blanc, Duck Confit with Brussels Sprouts and Mustard Sauce. In his cooking diary, he jotted down food preparation mistakes that needed correcting, reminding himself to pay attention to the neatness of his plates and avoid too much butter in the Trout Meunière. He scribbled the names of chefs he admired, a jumbled list of ingredients, an idea for a fundraiser. Another notebook contains a film treatment for "Shang: In the Eyes of the Dragon," with a road map for getting the movie in his head produced—a list of agents, producers, the addresses of the Screen Actors and Writers Guilds. After placing the files on a table in the backyard, Gloria closed the flaps on the box and shook her head.

Karen remembers her brother's exuberance and lust for life. His energy would always burn brightly at the beginning but eventually burst into flames. Looking back on it, that behavior now seems to his sister like the mania of bipolar disorder. In the late 1990s, Mark moved to New York City and lived with her and his niece, Avery, in Brooklyn. For the first several months, he added Technicolor to their quiet life. As he was getting settled into New York City, Mark volunteered at God's Love We Deliver, an organization that brings meals to people living with HIV/AIDS. Unlike her brother, Karen, a film editor, didn't like to cook, so Mark prepared and served meals and even threw dinner parties for her friends. "I had been living in that house ten years and never had a dinner party," she recalls. "But Mark was like, you buy, I'll fry. We'd shimmy together some tables, I'd invite my friends, and he'd make these really fabulous meals. It was super fun."

When it came time for Mark to get a job, he told his sister, "You start at the top." Mark bought a Zagat restaurant guide and started calling around, pitching himself to the city's four-star restaurants.

He didn't get a job at New York's No. 1 restaurant at the time, the Four Seasons, but Chanterelle, also four-star, hired him as a sous-chef after he volunteered to work for free for two weeks. He lasted almost two years. Mark told his sister, "I can get jobs and women. I can't keep them, but I know how to get them." Mark worked at more than two dozen restaurants throughout his life—from Chanterelle to McDonald's.

Mark's family and friends struggle to remember his downs. Like many of those who live with bipolar disorder, at first he hid the depression and later self-medicated with drugs. When the mania wore off, replaced by a depression that sapped his energy, creativity, joy, and spirit—the typical yin and yang of the disease—he created his own fix, chasing away the sadness with a drug high. His parents got a hint that Mark was suffering from some kind of depression after he left home to attend Chamberlayne Junior College in Boston in 1985. He made it a year. When Gloria and Ronald went to visit him, they found their son wasn't attending classes but sleeping all day.

It is clear that Mark did seek psychological help—over and over. In the files Gloria kept for her son, there are the names of several dozen mental health professionals who saw and treated Mark— psychiatrists, psychologists, social workers, and counselors—and many more names and numbers. Records from his jail stays show that Mark was receiving mental health treatment while incarcerated and at one point was taking medication for depression, Tourette's syndrome, and obsessive-compulsive disorder. At another point his distraught mother sought therapy, blaming herself for her son's condition.

Why didn't Mark's father, who studied behavioral science and eventually taught an undergraduate psychology class at Wesleyan, take a more active role in his son's mental illness? Gloria believes that her husband, who battled his way out of the Roxbury projects to earn his doctorate and secured a good job at a majority-white, elite college, simply didn't want to see what was happening with Mark. "Did his father get his undergraduate degree in psychology? Yes," says Gloria in her no-nonsense "pahk the cah" Boston accent. "Did he go to the national Association of Black Psychologists convention every year? Yes. Did he get psychiatric support for his son? No." Ronald passed away in 2019.

"God bless him," she continues quietly. "I think he didn't want his colleagues to know that his son had issues with addiction and needed psychiatric help. I think also, to be perfectly honest, we keep the emotions to ourselves in our family, but I guess I should've known."

Although the rate of those with bipolar disorder is the same for Black Americans as for other racial groups, the mental health condition can be significantly more dangerous for African Americans. Bipolar disorder, a brain condition that affects an estimated 2.3 million Americans, causes extreme shifts in mood, energy, and ability to function. These mood swings leave a person feeling very high—the manic phase—or low, the depressive phase. During mania, someone may experience excessive energy, increased activity, and a feeling of euphoria, as well as an inability to concentrate or sleep. These feelings heighten the chance of dangerous sexual behavior or use of drugs during this phase. It is during manic episodes that people may feel great bursts of creativity, and many of them balk at taking the mood-stabilizing medication necessary to control bipolar disorder, fearful that their creative impulses will be deadened. Depressive episodes are characterized by sadness, anxiety, pessimism, and hopelessness, as well as a loss of interest in pleasurable activities and difficulty concentrating. There may also be thoughts of death or suicide.

As potentially debilitating as bipolar disorder can be, it can be managed with psychotherapy and medication, allowing people to control their mood swings and lead fulfilling lives. Yet too often Black people are not diagnosed properly, leaving them without treatment. Research suggests that clinicians put more emphasis on manic than depressive symptoms in African Americans, which skews diagnoses toward schizophrenia even when these patients show similar symptoms as white patients. A 2014 study by University of California, Berkeley, researchers examined bipolar disorder treatment for Black and white Americans and found that Black people were misdiagnosed more often—typically with schizophrenia. Additionally, even with a proper diagnosis, Black people received less intensive treatment, leaving them less capable of leading stable and productive lives.

In Gloria McMullen's dusty boxes, she has dozens of files cataloging her son's attempts to kick his addiction to crack, his drug-related entanglements with law enforcement, and the money the family spent on rehab. Beginning in the late 1990s, Mark was in and out of drug rehabilitation—three stays for three weeks each at Rushford in Middletown and help at two facilities in other parts of Connecticut. He enrolled at Hazelden Betty Ford Foundation in Chicago and at St. Jude Retreats in Upstate New York. Despite addiction that was clearly severe, none of his seven stays in rehab lasted longer than just over a month. Money was at least part of the reason; rehab, medical bills, paying off drug debt, and other expenses related to Mark's substance abuse were draining his parents' savings. They spent at least several thousand dollars each time he received residential treatment; his longest stay, five weeks from May to July 2006 at the New York facility, cost his family $10,000.

Without question, Mark did not want to be an addict and was using drugs as his own form of medicine. He made a Herculean effort to recover. Between rehab stays, he attended Alcoholics Anonymous (AA) and Narcotics Anonymous (NA) meetings, and when he was incarcerated, Mark generally attended group and individual therapy. He left behind a handwritten paper trail of remorse, shame, and regret—journal entries, thank-you cards, apology notes, letters to judges and the parole board. In 2009, he tearfully told his mother, "I just want to be normal," begged forgiveness for his relapses, and thanked her for not giving up on him. That was also the year that Gloria McMullen created a recovery plan for herself. She attended meetings of Nar-Anon, a 12-step recovery program for friends and families of addicts. She wondered if she was an "enabler" and made a list of things that she would no longer do for her son, including give him money. She reminded herself that Mark was a drug addict and not in control. "I am not dealing with Mark, but the 'monster' within, 'the thing.'" She read up on Tough Love and looked into attending meetings. "Tough Love wasn't for me," says Gloria now. "I know a woman in Middletown who took the Tough Love approach, when her son was going through what Mark was going through."

She pauses. "I don't know if that would have made a difference, but her son is still alive, running a halfway house. My son is dead."

Black Americans who use drugs are disproportionately criminalized when they struggle with addiction. While Black adults in the United States use drugs at a rate about the same as or lower than their white counterparts, they are two and a half times more likely to be arrested for drug possession, per a 2016 joint study from Human Rights Watch and the American Civil Liberties Union. In Montana, Iowa, and Vermont, that disparity rises to more than six times; Minnesota, the epicenter of protests against policing in 2020, is right behind them, with Black adults nearly six times more likely to be arrested for drug possession than white adults.

That's not by accident and it's not new. In 1971, President Nixon fired the opening shots in the so-called war on drugs. It wasn't long before the national jail and prison population swelled from 300,000 to 2.3 million, with fully half the people incarcerated in federal facilities remanded on drug charges. The kicker: two-thirds of them were people of color, their lives interrupted by disproportionate policing. Perhaps the best way to observe the gap is to examine the ways people are prosecuted based on the drugs that fell them. In 1986, the Anti–Drug Abuse Act put in place sentencing known as the hundred-to-one cocaine-to-crack disparity, under which the distribution of five grams of crack—the less expensive form of cocaine associated with Black communities—carried a minimum sentence of five years. But someone, typically a white someone, would have to be caught with five hundred grams of cocaine before they would meet the same fate. Decades after the fact, Nixon's adviser John Ehrlichman disclosed that his administration intentionally used drug policy to vilify and criminalize Black people and quell protest. "We knew we couldn't make it illegal to be either against the war or black, but by getting the public to associate the hippies with marijuana and blacks with heroin, and then criminalizing both heavily, we could disrupt those communities," Ehrlichman said. "We could arrest their leaders, raid their homes, break up their meetings, and vilify them night after night on the evening news. Did we know we were lying about the drugs? Of course we did."

Little has changed when it comes to criminalization. While the 2010 Fair Sentencing Act reduced the disparity to eighteen to one—still a problem—the opioid crisis that plagues America has uncovered separate and unequal treatment for Black and white people suffering with addiction. The contradiction is stark. Where white people are offered sympathy and medical care and profiles in national newspapers, Black people are treated like criminals. It takes only a quick look at the news to see how the nation perceives the addicted. In fact, a 2017 analysis of the media found journalists running stories like "Painkiller Use Breeds New Face of Heroin Addiction," actively rebranding the narrative of addiction and sounding an alarm that people "just like us," presumably white and middle class, are suddenly at risk. In many of the stories highlighted by the report, Black Americans struggling with drug addiction are portrayed as people to fear and lock away. The events that led them to use drugs are downplayed in favor of whatever is deemed criminal about their behavior. Whites who abuse opioids are represented as victims of addiction whose lives are worthy of medical care and rehabilitation. Their life stories are laid out, the events that led to their downfall relayed as a cautionary—and redemptive—tale.

Federal spending also reveals unequal treatment: in 1986, as the crack epidemic surged, a quarter of the $1.74 billion in federal money tied to the Anti–Drug Abuse Act was set aside for programs that aimed to prevent drug use and treat patients; the rest was dedicated to enforcement and incarceration. But when it comes to opioids, the opposite is true: in 2018, 75 percent of the $7.4 billion congressional budget earmarked to respond to the opioid crisis had been set aside for treatment, and just 16 percent was earmarked for law enforcement.

In the fall of 2011, Mark swore again that he was going to turn his life around. This time his family allowed themselves to believe him. Five years earlier, in 2006, Gloria had taken her sister, their cousins, Karen, Chris, and Mark to Cape Verde, her father's homeland, to unite her American family with their African relatives. While there, Mark met Maria Santa, who worked as a cook for one of his Cape Verdean family members. He was intrigued by this beautiful woman with large eyes full of warmth and longing who spoke very little English, and she was captivated by the charming American man who loved to cook. After he returned home, Mark spent two years trying to get his new love, who goes by the name Kety, into the United States. Mark went to Senator Joe Lieberman, who eventually granted Kety a petition to immigrate. She married Mark in 2008 and in mid-July 2010, their son, Simon, was born. Fatherhood didn't heal Mark, but being a parent changed him. By all accounts, he was an enthusiastic, loving dad to Simon. In the first months of his son's life, Mark woke up early to give him baths, play with him, read to him, and take him to museums. He did the cooking, cleaning, and laundry to allow Kety time to grow into motherhood.

Still, his struggles with drugs and mental illness persisted. After he fell off the wagon and descended into a drug binge, he scribbled a note to Kety. "I do love you! I am sick. I am going to the doctor in Connecticut. I will be home tonight. Please be here. I am getting help. I need your help and support. By help, I mean every day."

In 2011, Mark was arrested for a parole violation. He begged to be placed in a diversionary program where he could receive intensive drug treatment and psychotherapy, attend 12-step meetings, and be attached to a system to monitor his psych meds. In a letter to the court, he wrote, "Since the birth of my son, I realized that I could make the world a better place and had resolved to do so. I intend to be the best possible roll [sic] model for my son on a daily basis. Showing him how to face problems and overcome them and how to live a life of service." Instead, Mark was sentenced to six months at Norfolk County House of Correction in Dedham, Massachusetts. During that time, he received no therapy or medication and resorted to doubling down by himself on a self-directed recovery program. He promised to take responsibility for his actions, wrote extensive lists of people from whom he should seek forgiveness—his wife, son, parents, and siblings at the top. He made financial restitution for his previous crimes and sketched out a drug relapse prevention plan.

A month after Mark's release, his mother planned the Labor Day family party. Generally, Gloria would drive her son to Boston, where he was staying at a Salvation Army halfway house, and then spend the night with her daughter-in-law and grandson in Quincy or circle back home. But after the family events, she didn't feel up to the two-hour-plus drive. Despite a nagging worry, she lent her son her husband's burgundy Hyundai. On September 6, Mark delivered Kety and Simon home safely, gave his son a bath, and cooked dinner for his wife, but never made it to the halfway house. The following day, Gloria McMullen received the news every mother dreads: your son is dead. The police didn't bother to let Kety know her husband had been killed; a close family friend drove to her house and delivered the news.

According to the police report and subsequent investigation, on Wednesday morning, September 7, two plainclothes Boston police officers patrolling an area of Roxbury known for drug activity saw Mark sitting in a car with a woman they said was a prostitute and drug user. When they approached the car, Mark drove away, leaving the woman behind. With guns pointed at him, he began a high-speed chase that involved dozens of both Boston and Massachusetts state police. He hit several police and other vehicles along the way until he ended up on a grass median at exit 14 of Route 3 in Rockland, nearly twenty miles from Roxbury. At that point, Mark was unarmed in the badly damaged Hyundai, with the airbag deployed, surrounded by about a dozen police cars and emergency vehicles. According to the official version, as Mark revved the engine, causing his tires to spin in the wet grass, Boston and state police officers approached his car. One of them, Christopher Carr, positioned himself in front of the Hyundai and, with his gun drawn, ordered Mark to stop. What the report says happened next makes little sense. Carr claims that Mark lurched his vehicle forward, in Carr's direction. He insists that Mark attempted to mow him down, and fearing for his life, Carr somehow managed to move from the front of the Hyundai to the driver's side and fire four times, hitting Mark in the arms and chest. Next—after Mark was shot (five times, according to the autopsy)—the official report becomes even stranger: "Mr. McMullen continued to physically resist and refused to comply with commands being issued by the officers. He was taken from the vehicle and after a struggle was handcuffed. At that point officers observed what appeared to be gunshots in Mr. McMullen's chest and neck area." Eventually, he was taken to South Shore Hospital and pronounced dead at 12:45 p.m.

The shocked and grief-stricken McMullen family disputed this official story, which common sense would assume was untrue. If Christopher Carr, standing in front of the Hyundai, feared for his life, how did he manage to move to the side of the car and kill Mark at point-blank range? If he was afraid of the lurching vehicle, why not shoot through the windshield—which was intact after the incident? Mark had been shot a number of times; how could he resist arrest and require handcuffs to be subdued? And why did the officers, who presumably had seen Carr shoot Mark—they were all standing there—only later "observe what appeared to be gunshots"? How could they not notice he was wounded and bleeding out?

Audrey Brianne has made a delicate peace with the mental illness she has lived with for so long. When she stepped back from styling to begin rehab, most of her clients understood she needed some time off, and she was able to keep her business's doors open with the help of assistants. As the entertainment industry recovers from the pandemic, her business is up and running, but she's clocking far fewer hours and servicing a smaller roster of clients. To maintain emotional balance, she belongs to a number of groups—AA, an alumni group from rehab, and a recovery circle of people who have experienced trauma. She says the camaraderie, accountability, and sharing of experiences steady her. She is an advocate for psychiatric medication and takes a cocktail of seven pills every morning. To fight the stigma surrounding mental health in the Black community, she is sharing her story. "When I discuss medication, I hear people say, 'That's white people talk,'" she says. "'You don't need all that medicine to feel okay. Just get some fresh air or pray on it.' But you can't pray depression away." When she goes deeper into her suicide attempt and describes the darkness of severe depression on podcasts and at events, she often strikes a chord in her audience. She says the positive feedback has been surprising, rewarding, and empowering.

Mark McMullen's story doesn't have a sunny ending. The Plymouth County DA's office conducted an investigation, determining that Mark had posed an immediate deadly threat to Carr and other officers, who were justified in killing him in cold blood. Seven months after the report and a year after Mark's death, the McMullens and activists held a rally in front of the Massachusetts State House in Boston, demanding justice. A flyer, with a smiling Mark holding Simon on his lap, asked, "Why Was Mark Shot?" In 2013, the Boston Police Department, apparently in an effort to derail the McMullen family's wrongful-death lawsuit, which was dragging through court, awarded Carr the department's highest honor, the Schroeder Brothers Memorial Medal, for the very incident that ended in the one-sided massacre of Mark McMullen.

Immediately following Mark's death, the McMullen family put in a request to get back the contents of the car he was murdered in. It took eight years for the police to respond. In January 2019, when the Massachusetts State Police finally released Mark's things, among the items was a copper recovery chip marking seven months of sobriety, a brochure with tips for staying clean and sober, a list of Cocaine Anonymous meetings in Maine, Massachusetts, and Rhode Island, and signed proof that he had attended weekly AA and NA meetings, the last one shortly before he died. Most heartbreaking, he had scrawled on a piece of paper torn from a yellow pad a note to his son, who was just over a year old at the time of his father's death. Mark had been incarcerated for Simon's first birthday and lost track of the note before he could deliver it. "You have successfully completed one year of life," Mark wrote, in all caps. "Congratulations, you've done a great job! You're on your way to a wonderful childhood. At this pace in one year, you will be two years old."

CHAPTER SEVEN

DISCRIMINATION AND ILL-TREATMENT CAN HARM EVERY BODY

On weekday mornings just before seven, a crowd gathers at the back entrance of the Friendship House, a drop-in center in Morgantown, West Virginia, that offers services and support for people dealing with mental health concerns and recovery from what it calls drug "misuse" in a state with a raging opioid drug crisis. On a rainy Tuesday in November 2020, about a dozen men and women—all white—wait at the door, which is situated in a parking lot across from Milan Puskar Health Right, the free health-care clinic for low-income uninsured or underinsured patients that runs the center. Another knot of people sit together on the pavement in front of a mural of Charlene Marshall, who became the first Black woman mayor in West Virginia when she won her election in Morgantown in 1991. The group huddles against the cold, swirls of cigarette smoke floating above them. They look gray and ground down, a sharp contrast to the brightly colored likeness of a full-bodied, smiling Marshall, who was barred from attending West Virginia University in the 1950s because the college banned Black students, but went on to serve seven years as mayor and another fourteen years in the West Virginia House of Delegates.

At seven on the nose, they are allowed to enter, and about a dozen people walk in. Some arrive empty-handed; others are freighted with their belongings, stuffed into suitcases and duffel bags they drag up the splintered stairs or in backpacks slung over their arms. One by one, they take a turn at the mustard-colored coffee urn, which looks like a relic from several decades ago. Morgan Anne Wood, a peer support specialist at the Friendship House, keeps up a stream of friendly chatter at the front desk, handing masks to those who aren't wearing them. Contracting COVID would make their fragile lives so much more tenuous. They cradle Styrofoam cups, clutching them like lifelines as they pull down their masks to take a sip of the strong coffee. Many of the visitors know each other, though others have just stumbled in from off the street, happy to find someplace warm and safe to sit for the next hour and a half, to get out of the cold and use the bathroom. They also come to Coffee Club to talk and exchange information, seeking out others who understand what it feels like to lose a job, a car, a home, and a family and end up on the street. And perhaps most important, others who understand the crater that psychiatric illness opens up, the pull of pills, meth, and heroin, and the downward spiral that often follows either.

Ashley and Jason turn their chairs to face each other. The two have just met and have become fast friends. Leaning in, their heads almost touching, they sit under a series of colorful paintings created by other Friendship House clients as part of an art therapy project. The piece directly above them reads, "Love Is Like a Flower. It Will Never Bloom Without Care," next to a bright orange tulip. Ashley's blond hair is cut in a neat bob. She's wearing a purple Champion sweat suit, the pants tucked into suede boots. A sturdy wool coat hangs on the back of her chair. She looks like Felicity Huffman, a star of the TV show *Desperate Housewives.* Jason wears glasses, sneakers, and dad jeans; he's clean-shaven, his hair also neatly cut. Together, they could be a suburban couple, volunteers, rather than clients.

Ashley, who is thirty-eight, has just landed in Morgantown, a city she liked when she was stationed there in 2006 while serving in the U.S. Army. She left the military the following year, returning to her hometown in western New York. There, she bought a house where she could raise her two young daughters. But then the trouble started. At first, she felt as if her home were getting sick. She describes it as vibrating. Then she worried that someone was following her, casing her home. At night, she could hear someone digging a tunnel under her house. She was diagnosed with PTSD, the result of being raped by several other soldiers while stationed at a base in Missouri. Eventually, her fears became overwhelming, and she felt so unsafe that she decided to run, leaving one daughter with her parents, the other with the girl's father. Ashley flew to Florida, bought a 2017 Toyota Highlander, and hit the road, staying in motels and shelters or sleeping in her car as she hopscotched between towns, cities, and states, living off her pension and military benefits. When she wrecked the car, she switched to the bus. She had landed in Morgantown the night before and secured a room in a motel but had a feeling she was being watched. So, she took a cab to another motel, where she ended up sleeping on a couch in the lobby until 5:00 a.m., when guests started waking up. Then she sat outside in the gazebo, until the doors of the Friendship House opened.

Jason is eager to help. He had a job as a carpenter earlier in the year, until an accident disabled his car and he could no longer get to work. He slept in his vehicle in the parking lot of a Walmart until it got too cold and he had spent the last of the $180 he had earned as a carpenter. The night before he joined Ashley and the others at Coffee Club, he slept at Bartlett House, a nonprofit shelter in Morgantown, funded by United Way. But because he got an emergency bed last night, he explains to Ashley, chances were slim he could get one again tonight. He pushes his glasses up with his index finger, looking like a roughed-up version of the college student he was ten years ago, before he dropped out.

People begin lining up in front of the Bartlett House emergency triage shelter just after sunset. When the doors open at 8:00 p.m., the crowd outside will jostle for one of about two dozen beds, and the rest are turned away. Those who don't get beds may head to Diamond Village, an encampment for the homeless in the Greenmont section of town, or curl up in an alley, under scaffolding, or on a bench. The other options that the Bartlett House offers, transitional and bridge housing, are reserved for families with children and young people aged eighteen to twenty-four. Many of the Bartlett

House clients are working poor in a town with an unemployment rate of 5.3 percent when I visited, which was lower than the state average. But the census points to a poverty rate of 33 percent. That means that most have jobs but are still too poor to survive on the state's $8.75 minimum wage. And it's even harder for people like Ashley, who struggles with mental illness, and Jason, who brings a criminal record left over from his younger days with him every time he applies for a job.

Jason isn't sure what he's going to do; Ashley either. She prefers sleeping in a shelter around other people who can protect her from her demons. But once she understands that Bartlett House isn't an option, she pulls a smartphone out of her orange leather purse and begins googling for a motel. As it nears the end of Coffee Club, the two leave together. Later, I see them walking from Trinity Episcopal Church, which serves free lunch to the homeless and hungry from its back door on Willey Street. They are part of a line of people shuffling the streets between the Friendship House and the church, like so many gray ghosts from a Dorothea Lange photograph.

The local government's annual Point-in-Time survey in January 2020 revealed that sixty-eight homeless individuals resided in Monongalia, the county that houses Morgantown, pre-COVID. But I have seen more than that between the Coffee Club, the free lunch program, and Diamond Village, though not every one of them is technically without a home. I pass Ashley and Jason again, still trying to figure out their sleeping arrangements, as they walk up Spruce Street carrying empty Styrofoam lunch containers. Across the street, the Alpha Phi house still has a sign announcing homecoming 2020. About a block up a steep hill, the University of West Virginia, a research institution with more than twenty-six thousand students and national-class sports teams, seems a world away. Improbably, Ashley has made up her face—foundation, blue eye shadow, mascara, and pink lipstick. She throws her lunch container in a trash bin and waves when I pass.

—

At its most basic, racism is defined as discrimination against a person or group of people because of race, resulting in harm and disadvantage. Its most pervasive and profound form, systemic or structural racism, is a set of power dynamics, braided into our country's history, culture, politics, and institutions, that reward white people while disadvantaging people of color, particularly African Americans. The system, which is invisible to most because it is so thoroughly baked into our experience, has created inequality in power, access, opportunity, treatment, policy, and outcomes.

Worst off are those at the intersection of race and poverty, and America punishes disadvantaged Black people with the least empathy, the most harm, and the fewest options. But our country judges all of the poor, including white people. U.S. culture overemphasizes personal responsibility, creating the false notion that poor Americans are largely to blame for their own poverty, with little interrogation of an unequal system that is beyond the control of the individual. People are poor as a result of their own laziness, immorality, and irresponsibility, the stereotype goes, and could turn their lives around by making better choices. America shames them by glorifying the privileged rich as well as Horatio Alger–esque examples of individuals who have overcome the odds, ignoring the societal barriers that create obstacles to health, wealth, well-being, and safety for many.

We have slowly been coming to grips with the bodily harm that discrimination has caused to Black people, who have struggled against mistreatment in various potent forms for centuries, across multiple generations. But discrimination is discrimination, and when sustained, it can cause harm to anybody, including white bodies. What if Black people are simply the canaries in the coal mine? In other words, what if the health disparities they have experienced aren't particular to the culture's view of Blackness, but are a result of the harm that oppression, neglect, and erasure can cause any body? The effects of discrimination may not look the same in white people from Appalachia as they do in Black women or other populations. But what if the wear and tear that comes with feeling that their world is collapsing and with battling against social and educational inequality is creating a similar outcome—homelessness, poor health, and early death?

That question sent me to West Virginia, where 93 percent of the population is white. West Virginia is part of Appalachia, the more than 200,000-square-mile region of the country made up of thirteen states—from southern New York to northern Mississippi. In the American imagination, the twenty-five million people of this region are all poor, white, uneducated, and backwoods, and like every stereotype this one is untrue. Still, the region is much less diverse than the country as a whole, and the economic distress is real: in the past several decades Appalachians have seen their wages stagnate, their jobs become obsolete, and their communities decay as a result of desertion or disinvestment by the companies that mined away their natural resources.

West Virginia is one of the whitest of all states and one of the most impoverished in the nation. It has among the country's highest unemployment and poverty rates for white people, as well as the overall lowest rate of labor force participation, 54 percent of working-age adults. Yet even that scorched-earth statistic understates the depth of the state's economic woes: it hides the large number of working poor who are barely scraping by on minimum wage, as well as the fact that many of the 46 percent who aren't currently part of the labor force would like to work but can't find jobs. It also leaves out people who want to work but have given up looking altogether. The coal industry, long the backbone of the economy, has extracted natural resources while leaving behind abandoned mines, shuttered businesses, depleted government coffers, black lungs, polluted land and water, and lost hopes and dreams. Mining jobs peaked at 125,000 in West Virginia in the 1940s, when the mines and the jobs they brought in paid enough to support families and scaffold the state's economy. When they began to close, as the industry became more automated and coal was replaced by other forms of energy produced in other states, the well-paying jobs left with them. By 2021, coal mining directly employed only about 13,000 West Virginians. Ironically, one of the poorest states has one of the richest governors: Jim Justice, himself a coal baron, who amassed billions. Along with Donald Trump, he promised to bring back coal and to loosen environmental and other regulations to make mining more profitable. That did little except to pile on dirty air, water, and soil into areas already overburdened with long-term pollution. In reality, the parts of West Virginia that for generations produced the most coal are now among the poorest communities in the state.

West Virginians have paid with their bodies. The state had the lowest life expectancy of any in the country when I was there; the average West Virginian could expect to live 74.4 years, according to 2018 data, compared with Hawaiians, the longest-lived Americans, at 81.3 years, or with the national average, which is 78.7 years. Racial health disparities still bubble up in a state with a Black population of less than 4 percent; on average Black West Virginians live several years less than white residents. Still, it is worth examining why early death in this overwhelmingly white state inched upward between 2010 and 2017, outstripping a broader downturn in life expectancy among white Americans. This, even though West Virginia expanded Medicaid in 2014, making access to health-care coverage more common for West Virginians than for Americans as a whole.

West Virginia is plagued by some of the same diseases that shorten the lives of Black Americans; poor physical health and mental health and the limitations in activity that result from those conditions are more prevalent in West Virginia than anywhere else in the nation. The obesity rate in West Virginia is nearly 40 percent, the highest in the nation. More than two-thirds of West Virginia adults are overweight or obese, raising the risk of heart disease, which is higher in the state than almost any place else in the United States. These health problems have been compounded by the slow drip of alcoholism, drug overdose, and suicide, which have reached crisis proportions, primarily among white Americans, in the past decade.

As with Black people, poor whites are generally blamed for their circumstances with little acknowledgment of the structural forces that stack the odds against so many. That conversation was raised a number of decibels by the author J. D. Vance, who used many of the same stereotypes usually foisted on Black Americans to describe the "broken" Appalachia that he fled. His 2016 best seller, *Hillbilly Elegy*, a bootstrapping story of the author's escape from rural Rust Belt Ohio into the arms of the coastal elite, zeroes in on welfare recipients gaming the government the same way Black so-called welfare queens have been accused of leeching off government largesse. The book—which came out in the middle of Donald Trump's frenzied run for president—became an explainer to understand poor and working-class whites, with Vance portraying the hillbilly culture as pathological, its members suffering from learned helplessness and appearing undeserving of sympathy.

In West Virginia, I am struck by the similarity to what W. E. B. Du Bois described when discussing the plight of Black people in the 1890s: the peculiar indifference to human suffering. When I meet Scott at the Friendship House, it takes a minute for him to stop shivering after spending the night on the street. Like Ashley, Jason, and the others, he has come to the Friendship House for a respite from the cold and rain, for the coffee, the company, and a bite to eat. He is hunkered down in a folding chair, alternately sipping coffee and slurping down a cup of ramen noodles, the noodles still hard because he's too hungry to wait for the hot water to soften them up. As is the case with many of the now two dozen people who will shuffle in and out of the room over the next hour and a half, his clothes are soiled and baggy, his oversized jeans pooling at his feet. He has a bushy gray beard, flecked with bits of noodle, and as he pulls down the hood of his sweatshirt, he rakes his long dirty nails through his matted hair. "I need a haircut," he says. His speech sounds slow and draggy. His left eye droops into a half-opened slit, making his right eye look wide with surprise. His left arm hangs limply at his side, and he keeps that hand stuffed in his pocket. We smile at each other and he tells me my hair is pretty, and I tell him his is too. He pulls down his mask to show me a snaggletoothed smile. Sizing up his eye and arm, the stiffness of his movements and pattern of speech, I guess he's had a stroke. "No," he explains. "An accident."

Scott, or Mr. Scotty as some of the others call him, is an Appalachia native, born and raised in Greene County, Pennsylvania, just over the northern border of West Virginia. In 1993, he was working at a tire shop when he was involved in a car accident that killed a friend and put Scott in a coma for three months. After he regained consciousness, his injuries were so severe that he required a wheelchair and later physical therapy to relearn to walk and talk. Once mobile and partially recovered, Scott was arrested for the role he played in his friend's death. His memories are hazy, and the sequence of his life after the accident and release from prison remains jumbled because of the permanent effects of the head injury. As he struggles to recount where he has lived and how he has survived in the more than twenty-five years since the accident, I interrupt to ask him his age, sizing him up to be about seventy. "I'm forty-eight," he says.

Immediately I think of weathering. Though most of her research has centered on Black-white health disparities, more recently Arline Geronimus has expanded her theory of weathering to other disadvantaged groups who are the targets of sustained discrimination. Several years ago, Nicole Novak, one of her doctoral students, led her to Postville, Iowa. There, in May 2008, about 900 federal immigration officials in SWAT gear stormed onto the factory floor of a large meat processing plant to arrest 389 employees, most from Guatemala. Suspected of being undocumented, the men and women were handcuffed, linked by chains at the waist, herded into buses with blacked-out windows, and held in detention centers. Families were ripped apart, and some people, including children without their parents, sought refuge in the local Catholic church.

Novak, who is from Iowa, took Geronimus's class Structural Influences on Health and Social Behavior at the University of Michigan School of Public Health in 2012. As a final assignment, Geronimus asked her students to describe a public health issue and think about it through a structural lens. Novak wrote about the Postville raid. Geronimus was both outraged and intrigued and asked Novak to work with her to examine birth outcomes in the years before and after the raid. The two spent more than a year nudging the Iowa Department of Public Health for data from all 209,389 births in

Iowa from 2006 to 2010. They also combed Spanish-language newspapers, collecting articles about the raid and its aftermath. These included alarming eyewitness accounts and frightening images from Postville that spread throughout Latinx communities in Iowa via the press. Rumors of impending raids and ICE going door to door panicked people throughout the state.

Ultimately, Geronimus, Novak, and another colleague, Aresha M. Martinez-Cardoso, found that for the nine months after the Postville incident, Latinx mothers—both U.S.-born and immigrant—had a 24 percent higher risk of delivering a low-birth-weight baby than before the raid. Most of these Latinx mothers across Iowa who gave birth to underweight babies weren't directly connected to the Postville crackdown and most lived far away from the town. Yet many of them still experienced enough fear, anxiety, and trauma to create a weathering effect on their bodies. This was associated with lower birth weight, even after controlling for age, smoking, and other factors. The study, published in 2017 in the *International Journal of Epidemiology*, served as a dangerous omen of the toll on the health of Americans that could be taken by the cruel methods of Donald Trump's immigration policies.

If Black and Latinx people can have their health eroded by stress caused by ill-treatment, what about white people like Scott? His Sisyphean coping in the face of dire life circumstances seemed to age him. Those circumstances went beyond the consequences of his accident. A high school dropout, Scott grew up in an area of Appalachia where secure jobs dried up and the poverty rate crept to 20 percent. He was already hanging by a thread before disability and incarceration derailed his life. Scott's circumstances are clearly extreme. But many of the people shuffling up and down the streets of Morgantown between the Friendship House, the back door of Trinity Church, Bartlett House, and Diamond Village seemed weathered by life's headwinds. Though the experiences of Blacks and Latinx Iowans don't match exactly with white West Virginians, the people I see in Morgantown are suffering because the bottom has fallen out of their lives and their tenacious efforts to hang on have made them look and seem older than their biological ages would suggest.

Caitlin Sussman, the Friendship House's program director, keeps a scrapbook of clients who haven't managed to weather life's storms. The front of the white binder reads, "In Loving Memory of Our Past Loved Ones," with rainbows splashed to the sides. Sussman, who was raised in rural Maryland an hour east of Morgantown and graduated from the University of West Virginia's social work school, thumbs through page after page of mostly young and middle-aged white men and a few women. Charles Ray Cress died in 2014 at age forty. He loved fishing and hunting; in his tribute photo, he poses with his hands wrapped around the antlers of a deer he has just shot. Charles Lee Shultz stares directly into the camera; he looks tired and slightly annoyed. He loved country music and karaoke before he passed away in 2016 at the age of fifty-six. Charles Ellis Everett died the same year at fifty-three. He smiles in a snapshot taken at sunset, his fishing rod extending over a favorite lake. Jason Allen Smith died the same year at age thirty, leaving behind two daughters and a son. The following year, Kenny Allen Johnson passed away at fifty-one; his father and two brothers had proceeded him in death. In 2019, Etta Pearl Saint, a big-boned redhead, died just before her fiftieth birthday. Her boyfriend, Clay, wrote in the book, "She was my partner, friend and lover. She will always be my angel." Sussman explains that these people have died from a variety of causes—heart disease, diabetes, cancer, suicide, alcoholism, and drug addiction. She pauses when she lands on a picture of Phil McCarty, a volunteer at the Friendship House who had died a few months before. He's wearing a mask and foggy horn-rimmed glasses and holding a certificate celebrating his volunteer work with the homeless during the pandemic. A few months later, after being clean for a year and a half, he relapsed and died of a heroin overdose at age forty-one.

Each of these men and women adds to the grim accounting of what have been labeled deaths of despair. Nearly every U.S. media outlet covered the 2015 study by Anne Case and Angus Deaton that pointed to the rising rate of deaths among white Americans in their mid-forties to mid-fifties between 1999 and 2013. The married Princeton economists blamed this death rate among whites—not seen since the height of the AIDS epidemic—on suicide, drug overdoses, and alcoholic liver disease, particularly in states such as Arkansas, Kentucky, Mississippi, and West Virginia. The researchers noted declines in self-reported health, mental health, and ability to work, increased reports of pain, and deteriorating liver function, which they believed pointed to growing midlife distress almost entirely among white Americans without four-year college degrees.

The drug overdose numbers are most alarming. The rate of opioid overdose has drastically increased nationally, and West Virginia is at the epicenter with the country's highest rate of overdose deaths. The sad statistics of West Virginia and Appalachia as a whole have been clouded by the belief that poverty and unemployment stem from laziness and bad personal choices and that the addiction that can follow results from weakness and lack of willpower. This contradicts the reality that pharmaceutical companies aggressively marketed OxyContin as a safe pain pill. Between 1997, just after Purdue Pharma released OxyContin to the market, and 2007, prescriptions for opioid medication skyrocketed 402 percent in the United States. But in 2007, the government cracked down on Purdue Pharma, which meant that buying opioid medication on the street became more difficult and much more expensive. Those who had gotten hooked on prescription medication filled the void with cheaper and more dangerous heroin and fentanyl, a synthetic opioid. The vast majority of heroin users, studies show, first used prescription medication. Though Purdue Pharma pleaded guilty to charges of misleading regulators, doctors, and patients about the drug's risk of addiction and potential for abuse, the personal responsibility narrative remains stubbornly alive.

Race runs through this problem in complicated ways. Some in the field believe Blacks have avoided the brunt of the opioid crisis because physicians, falsely believing African Americans have superhuman pain tolerance, prescribed pain medication to them less frequently. This myth, left over from slavery, might have inadvertently prevented tens of thousands of Black overdose deaths, though it also might have resulted in undocumented suffering for those who were undermedicated for a variety of health concerns—from broken bones to cesarean sections. Other myths about Black people—that they were more likely to become addicted to drugs or to sell them—might have also led to fewer prescriptions written for pain medication.

The opioid epidemic is drenched in the kind of shame and judgment that leads to deaths and diseases of despair. Geronimus, while acknowledging the numbers and the problem, warns away from the term "of despair," which suggests passivity and a kind of giving up. Instead, similar to the way she describes how weathering affects the bodies of Black and brown people, Geronimus connects the falling life expectancy in white Americans to high-effort coping that is softly killing those who are working doggedly against barriers and difficulties to survive. These are people who believed that hard work was enough to create good lives and also internalized the opposite: that those who failed didn't work hard enough or suffered from a character defect. There is not enough acknowledgment in their communities that the economy had changed in ways that make it more difficult than in the past for people with the least education to find and keep jobs. This disconnect creates emotional distress and erodes physical health.

Despite Geronimus's dislike of the term, despair seems etched into the faces of those people who live in Diamond Village, an encampment that has turned into a shelter of last resort for people in Morgantown. Many of those who have made their homes in the chaotic jumble of tents, situated on a parcel of public land down the hill from Pennsylvania Avenue next to Deckers Creek, seem to have gotten tired of battling life's barriers and have sunk into hopelessness. Many are the Americans whom Case and Deaton describe as "drinking themselves to death, or poisoning themselves with drugs," or, at rock bottom, "shooting or hanging themselves." Their belongings, strewn on the ground among the tents, tell the stories of lost lives: yellowed storage bins, a rake and mop stuck in a shopping cart, a wheelchair tipped on its side, a milk crate full of rusted pots and pans, a yoga mat, a cracked kiddie pool, a printer, a space heater, a brown velour pullout couch, and a Persian rug draped over a sagging clothesline.

Dani Ludwig, a peer recovery coach at the Friendship House, walks comfortably through Diamond Village. She steps around a fire pit, making her way to the back of the collection of tents, calling out, "Who's here?" She stops to point to a makeshift garden, vegetables planted in blue, green, and red storage bins. Over the summer, it produced peppers, carrots, cucumbers, and squash, but as winter approaches, one lone green tomato clings to a tangle of vines. Ludwig, who has three piercings in her nose, a fuzzy buzz cut, and a tattoo of Maleficent on her leg, feels at home in what seems like human chaos. She connects with the people who live inside the tents because she's been there: Seventeen years of active drug addiction—except for the nine months she was pregnant with her daughter, Olivia—meant that she spent several years, off and on, living in a tent city like this one in another part of West Virginia. She stripped and did sex work to survive and dug through dumpsters at the back door of Little Caesars and Food Lion to eat. Her mother was so alarmed by her daughter's descent that she bought her a cemetery plot and told her, "This is where I'm going to put you."

In December 2017, she was both using and selling heroin when an acquaintance called and asked her if he could buy from her. Ludwig met her friend in the parking lot of a 7-Eleven and sold him $90 worth of heroin; that fix killed him three days before Christmas. Ludwig was arrested on felony charges and incarcerated for six months. She refused bond—too afraid of either catching another charge on the outside or dying of an overdose. Eventually, she was able to persuade a social worker to help her into rehab, and her sentence was reduced. In 2018 she ended up in Sober Living, a program in Morgantown that provides housing and support for people dealing with addiction as they reintegrate back into the community. In 2019, drug-free, she began working for the Friendship House, and a year later she was reunited with Olivia.

Her eyes sweep over the back end of the encampment, several yards from a three-story house with dirty siding and boarded-up windows, where Daniel is sitting on his haunches in front of his tent eating what looks like cereal out of a paper bowl. He is wearing an oversized Drippin Swag T-shirt stained with old food and is surrounded by a dolly, a portable storage bin containing three onions, a pile of empty plastic soft drink bottles, and, improbably, a Christmas tea towel. He moved into Diamond Village four months ago, from an abandoned house up the street where he had been squatting. Raised in Morgantown, he dropped out of school in ninth grade and got a job as a welder. He lost that job and struggled to find another. As is the case for many of the least educated Americans, his opportunities were few. He started buying pills off the street, grinding them up, and snorting them to feel the high faster. Though prescriptions for pain meds began to fall across the country that year, some areas of West Virginia continued to be inundated with them. But after a big bust in Morgantown about five years later, supplies dried up. The price of Perc 30s—Daniel's drug of choice, which contain a thirty-milligram dose of oxycodone—went from $15 a piece to $50. So he switched to heroin, which was much cheaper. His long-standing addiction shows: his body is covered with scabs where he injects drugs, even on his face and ears, some of them bloody. He has a girlfriend who is incarcerated and a son and daughter he hasn't seen in years. If he closes his eyes very tight, he can remember his children's faces, but otherwise he doesn't think about them—or his life or his future.

Paula, a friendly blonde wearing a blue sweatshirt and turquoise jewelry, walks by with a black garbage bag, picking up trash. She has a leather tote slung over her arm and shifts it slightly as she leans down to feed a Vienna sausage to Pedro, the camp cat, before she continues tidying up. Paula grew up in Morgantown and graduated from the University of West Virginia, just up the hill, with a degree in psychology, a minor in criminal justice. Now forty-nine, she was married for twelve years and has two adult children and a grandchild. Before she ended up in Diamond Village, she was running her own business, doing remote customer service for companies like Quicken. She looks up from her hands. "I know you're wondering what the hell happened, right?

"I'm bipolar," she explains. "I love the manic phases but hate the lows. It's not like being depressed or sad. It's a deep hopelessness like nothing you could ever imagine."

Medication never worked for her. It made her feel dead inside. To avoid the crushing lows, she self-medicates with crystal meth. Even while using "ice," she managed to maintain her business, living in a house in Morgantown with friends. But in March her computer was hacked, and she couldn't get her files back up, which meant the end of her business. About a month later, someone died in the apartment below them, and the landlord evicted anybody whose name wasn't on a lease. She had only a few hours to pack up before a sheriff came to the property. After bouncing around, couch surfing, for a few months, she claimed a tent in Diamond Village.

"At first to me, it just looked like tents on top of each other," she says. "But now it feels more like home." She describes family meals and sitting around the fire pit with other Diamond Village residents. Unlike Daniel, Paula can see a future for herself. Eventually, she'd like to restart her business or renew her social work license and find a job as a caseworker of some sort. A thick paperback with a light blue cover is sticking out of the top of her bag. She's reading *Broken Open: How Difficult Times Can Help Us Grow.*

Ludwig gives Paula and Daniel each a bottle of water and several doses of Narcan, a nasal spray containing naloxone, a drug used to counteract the life-threatening effects of an opioid overdose. In the nine months Diamond Village had been open, a hundred overdoses had been reversed there using the drug, and no one had died. Several hours after I walk through, however, the first person does die at the encampment. On October 27, 2020, police found Rebecca Colgan, a young Black woman I didn't see when I visited with Ludwig, lying on her back with a used needle filled with fresh blood next to her body. A month later, the City of Morgantown shut down Diamond Village.

The day after Rebecca Colgan was found dead, I was scheduled to meet with volunteers from SOAR (Solutions Oriented Addiction Response), a harm-reduction group in Charleston, West Virginia's capital and largest city. Charleston has been in the grip of a raging opioid addiction crisis since pharmaceutical companies began inundating the area with prescription pain meds. Between 2007 and 2012, drug wholesalers flooded West Virginia with 780 million hydrocodone and oxycodone pills, according to the Pulitzer Prize–winning reporting of Eric Eyre of the *Charleston Gazette-Mail.* All told, these shipments—mainly to counties in the southern part of the state surrounding the capital—amounted to 433 pain pills for every man, woman, and child in West Virginia, according to Eyre's reporting. In response, law enforcement cracked down on pain management clinics, doctors, and "pill mill" pharmacies. As prescription opioids dried up, people turned to injecting heroin and fentanyl, often using and sharing needles and syringes. This led to an outbreak of HIV in southern West Virginia, similar to a well-documented cluster of cases tied to IV drug use in rural Scott County, Indiana, in 2014 and 2015. West Virginia has historically had low rates of HIV cases, but parts of the state have turned into HIV epicenters.

In 2015, worried officials at the Kanawha-Charleston Health Department brought a syringe exchange to Charleston. Several decades of research from all over the United States and the world provides crystal-clear evidence that syringe exchange programs are safe and effective. These programs have also been shown both to save money and to create opportunities for people to get into treatment and care.

Despite the abundance of data about the benefits of this kind of harm reduction, syringe exchange advocates are often met with suspicion, accused of encouraging drug use and promoting crime. Those fears mounted in Charleston and came to a head in 2018 when the program could not meet the needs of the number of people looking to exchange dirty syringes and "points" or "sharps," words that describe needles, for clean ones. At its peak, nearly five hundred drug users passed through the exchange in just eight hours—in a city of fewer than fifty thousand people. The mayor at the time, Danny Jones, called the syringe exchange program a "mini-mall for junkies and drug dealers." The city shut it down that year, leaving Charleston with only a much smaller exchange run by a private clinic.

As HIV and overdoses spiked among injection drug users, SOAR was created to fill the void of government response. Largely under the radar, harm-reduction volunteers launched a DIY street outreach syringe exchange project in the parking lot of Unitarian Universalist Congregation (UUC), a progressive church at the corner of Vine Street and Kanawha Boulevard. Every other Wednesday evening, they collect used needles and syringes and exchange them for clean, sterile ones. They also offer food, water, HIV tests, condoms, and hundreds of doses of Narcan to as many as three hundred people who come through each night. As I was packing for the two-and-a-half-hour drive south from Morgantown to Charleston to observe the work, Joe Solomon, one of SOAR's organizers, emailed me. The group was considering canceling the week's Wednesday night event after a local television reporter called attention to its work with a lurid, tabloid-style story. The spot included hazy video recorded on the sly by an unnamed woman who said she had received sixty needles from SOAR over two visits without turning in any needles or syringes. The "exclusive investigation" takes credit for alerting the police to SOAR's activities. In the end, Solomon and the other volunteers decided to lie low and not hand out syringes but still conduct HIV testing and distribute Narcan and other supplies.

By the time I arrive, the sun is setting and people are beginning to stream into the parking lot at UUC. Solomon, wearing foggy glasses and a black mask that says, "I Save Lives," stands in front of a table groaning with supplies. He spends most of his time apologizing as he breaks the bad news that there are no syringes and points tonight.

Behind him an assembly line of volunteers, including two ministers from the church, collect "returns," or syringes, in white plastic canisters and sharps in a red medical waste container. Hands sheathed in blue surgical gloves, they also distribute masks, hygiene wipes, water, Pop-Tarts, snack bags of Goldfish, granola bars, tampons, condoms, and blankets donated by another church. At another table, a nurse hands out naloxone and offers wound care. A young couple—a man in baggy fatigues pushing a woman in a wheelchair—approaches Solomon. Her head is slumped over, stringy blond hair brushing a dirty backpack on her lap. Joe shakes his head and says he's sorry. Their faces show less despair than desperation. Before he wheels her away, the man grabs a snowy-white blanket from the pile and stuffs it in the backpack. Another couple approaches Solomon, this time older, although I've learned to stop guessing anyone's age anymore. Their eyes are flinty, their hands jittery as they inquire about "sharps." When Solomon apologizes—again—and suggests HIV testing and counseling offered by the city's Ryan White program, they stomp off. They pass a woman pushing a shopping cart full of her belongings; the man catches her eye. "They ain't got nothing here. Just for HIV," he spits at her over his shoulder. She turns, puts her feet on the shopping cart, and rides it out of the lot. Another man, wearing a Pittsburgh Steelers cap and matching yellow and black hoodie, approaches the table. "So, you don't have any needles?" "No, I'm sorry," Solomon tells him, and offers him Narcan. "You sure you don't have any clean ones?" the man insists, grabbing Solomon's sleeve. He shakes his head. "I need some bad, man," the man says.

I go to the back and sign up for an HIV test so that I can see how the process works and talk to a provider. After my OraQuick blood test, as I wait for my results, a woman with hair dyed the color of dark cherries sits down next to me. She's in line behind me for results. She looks agitated, her leg is shaking erratically, and the cigarette in her hand is quivering. Between puffs, she gnaws at the Band-Aid on her fingertip. "You are waiting for your test?" she asks me. I tell her yes. "You, too?" "Yeah," she says.

She explains that she used to get points from the health department, but once the exchange ended, clean syringes and needles
became hit-or-miss. A friend told her about SOAR, but when she
showed up tonight, she learned that the exchange had been disabled.
"To be honest, I been sharing, had no choice," she explains. "I'm
scared I got it," she says, and I understand that she means HIV. As
we wait, Chrissy, a peer recovery support specialist, approaches us.
She asks if we want cigarettes; the woman with the burgundy hair
takes one from her. Chrissy hands her a business card from a local
drug recovery program and explains that she was an active user for
half her life. "You can get help," she says. The woman stuffs the card
into the pocket of her jacket, takes a drag on the cigarette, and says
thank you. Chrissy moves on, approaching two young women on
Sting-Ray bicycles who look like sisters, pulling more business cards
out of her fanny pack.

When my number is called, the burgundy-haired woman wishes
me luck. I come out of the tent and give her a thumbs-up and hand
her the $10 gift card and $5 Kroger card I received in exchange for
testing. I ask her to let me know how it goes as her number is called
and she stands up. On this evening, many fewer people come by
SOAR. Solomon explains that news spread fast about the TV report
and people were afraid the police would raid the event. He estimates
that only about seventy have come through, down from several hundred on an average night. At one point, a blond woman wearing
sunglasses and spotless white workout clothes climbs out of a Jeep
SUV. Another organizer, Brooke Parker, points her head toward the
woman and whispers something to Solomon. They both watch her,
worried that she's a television reporter, as she walks across the parking lot with her head down, carrying a white canister. She leaves the
used points and syringes at the returns table. "She's just dropping off
for family, I guess," says Parker as the woman gets back in the Jeep
and drives away.

That evening, the Ryan White providers administered thirty-four
HIV tests. Three people test positive; usually they record one, two
at most. I think about the woman with the burgundy hair. About

twenty minutes after she snubs out her cigarette to learn her test results, I see her rush out of one of the three HIV counseling tents. She's moving too fast for me to catch her. The sun is almost completely set, and under a streetlight I see her shove her hands into her jacket pockets and walk hurriedly into the night.

CHAPTER EIGHT

PUTTING THE CARE BACK IN HEALTH CARE: SOLUTIONS

In 1986, I was assigned to write about HIV/AIDS, then still known as gay-related immunodeficiency disease, or GRID, for *Essence* magazine. No one knew much about this mysterious disease except that it struck gay men and people who injected drugs. I was such a novice writer that I was surprised to receive this major assignment. I later found out that several more seasoned writers had turned it down, afraid of "catching" the scary virus that was a death sentence for a growing number of people.

As part of my reporting, I went to the Bronx to interview a woman who had contracted the disease from her boyfriend, who had been addicted to heroin. Holding her nineteen-month-old daughter on her lap, she described the puzzling symptoms that had begun several months earlier. She was tired and had been losing more and more weight. I could see that her brown skin had a grayish tint, and she could barely hold up her head. I set my notebook aside and took the toddler from her as she continued to talk. The impish little girl, her hair in two fuzzy pigtails, looked at me and showed a gummy smile, and I saw that her mouth was lined with something white and furry.

Because of my inexperience as a medical journalist, our editor in chief paired me with her college biomedicine professor to walk me through the science of the illness. When I described the baby's mouth to her, she identified the condition as a fungal infection called thrush, common among people with GRID. At that moment, I understood that this virus was eating away at both the woman and her daughter. By the time the story ran in the June 1987 issue of the magazine with the headline "Nobody's Safe," both the mother and her baby girl were dead.

Mine was apparently the first reported article about HIV/AIDS for an ethnic publication. It received praise and recognition and opened the eyes of many to HIV and its impact on African Americans, and it generated promises from Black leaders to take action. This piece also marked the moment I realized that these kinds of stories would be my life's work. I had a responsibility to continue to use the knowledge I had gained to keep covering this disease. I wrote or edited several more articles on AIDS and also volunteered with the Black AIDS Institute to teach other journalists of color to report and write about the virus. Because I'm an optimist, I assumed there would soon be an end to this terrible plague, and my work, in this area at least, would be finished.

Sure enough, in 1996, scientists discovered a lifesaving "cocktail" of highly active antiretroviral drugs that could stop HIV in its tracks. With this new treatment, thousands of people experienced the Lazarus effect and were brought back from near death, and the AIDS mortality rate plummeted. In November 1996, a *New York Times Magazine* cover story, "When Plagues End," announced that AIDS no longer equaled death but merely illness. A month later, *Newsweek* asked, "The End of Aids?" Despite overall good news, the answer was actually no; the plague wasn't over. Just as America was celebrating the end of AIDS, the virus grabbed hold of Black America. HIV had been framed primarily as a gay white disease, but in 1996 for the first time Blacks accounted for a larger proportion of AIDS cases (41 percent) than whites, and HIV/AIDS became the leading cause of death for all Black Americans aged twenty-five to forty-four. This information remained underreported outside Black media. I left *Essence* to work at *The New York Times,* where I continued to cover AIDS, but found it challenging to get articles into the paper because the epidemic was supposed to be over in America. My friend and colleague Lynette Clemetson, another Black woman who was reporting for the *Times,* out of Washington, D.C., and I fought our skeptical editors to do a package about the AIDS epidemic in Black America. We got the go-ahead, and two of my stories made it to the front page of the *Times* in 2004. The first, "AIDS Fears Grow for Black Women," reported that Black women were the fastest-growing group of newly infected and that the South was hardest hit. The second, "Patients with H.I.V. Seen as Separated by a Racial Divide," argued that even as others lived with HIV/AIDS as a "manageable" illness, Black people continued to die from it in disproportionate numbers. Both of these stories generated recognition about the disease in Black Americans, as my "Nobody's Safe" piece had, and promises by authorities to do better. I, again, assumed there would soon be an end to this plague and my work would be finished.

In 2016, now nearly thirty years after my initial *Essence* article, twenty years after the plague was pronounced dead, and more than a decade after my two major HIV stories for the *Times,* I learned that if trends held, half of all Black gay and bisexual men would be living with HIV within their lifetimes. The virus was still most active in southern states, which accounted for more than half of all new HIV diagnoses; southern cities had the highest prevalence of HIV among queer Black men (and transgender women). Ground zero was Jackson, the capital of Mississippi, our most impoverished state. The South also had and has the highest numbers of people living with HIV who didn't know they had been infected, which meant they were not engaged in lifesaving treatment and care and were at risk of infecting others. An unconscionable number of them were dying: among Black men in this region, the death rate from an HIV-related cause was seven times higher than for the U.S. population at large.

I spent half a year reporting in Jackson and retracing the history of HIV/AIDS in America to understand how Black people had, once again, been left behind. I was haunted by the memory of the young dying mother in the Bronx when I visited Jordon, a college kid living in small-town Mississippi who had contracted HIV in 2016. He was bedridden, and his skin had that same ghostly gray pallor. Sweatpants pooled around his stick-thin legs, so fragile you could snap them in two. Though this was the rural South in 2016, he looked as if he were trapped in a time warp that had carried him to the New York City of 1986.

The story, which ran on the cover of *The New York Times Magazine* in June 2017, was called "America's Hidden H.I.V. Epidemic." Though this epidemic wasn't hidden, except in plain sight, the most common response to the article was shock, given that the plague had supposedly ended. I heard more promises to do better.

At this point, in 2021, I am starting to wonder if there ever will be an end to this plague. When exactly is my work going to be over? And this is not just true of HIV. In 1991, I wrote a story for *Essence* called "Showdown at Sunrise" that looked at environmental racism through the experience of a community in Cancer Alley, the eighty-five-mile stretch of the Mississippi River known for its cluster of polluting petrochemical manufacturers. Sunrise, a town in southeastern Louisiana, had been founded by enslaved people, and their descendants were being poisoned by proximity to a knot of oil and chemical companies.

Nearly thirty years later, I wrote "The Refinery Next Door," which looked at the same problem, this time through the lens of a Black community in Philadelphia that had been situated next to the largest and oldest refinery on the East Coast. This story, which ran in *The New York Times Magazine* in August 2020, also highlighted a community of Black people suffering from clusters of cancer, retold some of the same history of the environmental justice movement, and even featured some of the same experts. I discovered that the problem had actually worsened in the nearly three decades since I first covered it and that Black Americans were more likely to be situated near polluting facilities than in previous decades. Also in 1991, I wrote an *Essence* story called "Emergency: Crisis in Our Healthcare," which sounded the alarm about racial disparities in medical treatment and care. Exactly thirty years later, I used that article as background for the introduction to this book, noting how little progress our country has made in coming up with lasting solutions to this long-standing crisis. And now, as I write, the COVID-19 pandemic, which I discuss in the afterword, is the latest embodiment of the issues I've been writing about for so long. Viruses like HIV and COVID as well as other diseases strike discriminately at marginalized communities, grasping at patterns of inequality and sinking into the fault lines of our society.

As I have laid out, the reasons for racial health disparities are threefold: long-standing discrimination in the institutions and structures of American society that has harmed and continues to harm Black communities, making them less "healthy"; racism in society that wears away the bodies of Black people and those from other groups who are treated poorly; and bias in health care that creates a system of unequal treatment. It will be difficult to turn around the health of Black communities, burdened as they are by a history of systemic racism. It will take even longer to upend societal racism and stop its destructive effects. Putting an end to racism in health care, while easier to see and solve, is also years away.

But still, I remain optimistic and trust that the lessons we learn from this work will inform how our society addresses other communities as well, whether they are poor whites in West Virginia or terrorized Latinx in Postville, Iowa. I feel hopeful when I look at my previous articles on racial health disparities and see a common through line: committed, determined people who are wrapping their arms around individuals and communities in order to unravel some of America's most entrenched health problems. I am also encouraged by the growing recognition that racism in medical care has long existed and continues to cause harm: I see medical societies, universities, hospitals, and other institutions, organizations, and individuals grappling with it and working to do better. I am also inspired by medical students, the health-care providers of the future, who want to be better and do better.

One of these committed, determined people is Cedric Sturdevant. In 2016, while working on my article about HIV in Mississippi, I met Cedric, a project coordinator at My Brother's Keeper, a nonprofit community health organization in Jackson. He functioned in the improvised role of visiting nurse, motivational coach, and father figure to a growing number of young Black gay and bisexual men and transgender women suffering from or at risk for contracting HIV/AIDS. I spent several weeks with him, off and on, as he made his rounds along the bumpy streets and back roads of Jackson in a thirteen-year-old Ford Expedition with cracked seats, chipped paint, and a bumper sticker that said, "Mean People Suck." Without Sturdevant, it was clear that many of his clients would not get to the doctor appointments, pharmacies, food banks, and counseling sessions that can make the difference between life and death.

Negotiating a maze of unpaved roads in West Jackson, I was with him when he dropped off HIV medication at the home of a couple, one HIV-positive, the other HIV-negative, in the neighborhood locals call the Bottom, where every fifth or sixth home is abandoned, windows are broken, doors hang off the hinges, and downed limbs and dry leaves blanket front yards. Sturdevant banged on the door of a small house, its yard overgrown with weeds; he knew not to leave the package on the doorstep, where it could be stolen. After a while a young man emerged, shirtless, shrugging off sleep. He had just gotten out of jail. Sturdevant handed him the package, shook his hand, and told him, "Stay out of trouble."

Sturdevant drove on another fifteen minutes to pick up a teenager, still reeling from the HIV diagnosis he had received earlier that year. As they headed to and from a doctor's appointment and a meeting with a counselor, Sturdevant, slow talking and patient, with eyes that disappeared into his cheekbones when he smiled and a snowy beard, gently grilled him, reminding him to stay on his meds. The teen slumped in the backseat, half listening, half checking his texts. He looked up briefly when Sturdevant told him, "You've come a long way. I'm proud of you." The young man barely said goodbye as he jumped out of the car in front of a convenience store on an avenue scattered with a pawnshop, a liquor store, and several Baptist churches. He all but admitted he was planning to spend the afternoon smoking weed and looking at Instagram. "Knucklehead,"

Sturdevant whispered as the teen slammed the door. Pulling off his favorite Dallas Cowboys baseball cap and running a hand over his bald head, Sturdevant added softly, "Breaks my heart."

Sturdevant is homegrown. He was born and raised in Metcalfe, a tiny town in the Mississippi delta. He understands all too well the fear, stigma, and isolation that can come with being a Black gay man in the South. When he was diagnosed with HIV in 2005, Sturdevant knew little about the virus and was too depressed and ashamed to tell anyone at first. When his partner died the following year, he let the disease consume him. With a fever of 103, he was so weak and sick he couldn't keep water down. Sturdevant has shared his story too many times to count, to let young men know that he's been there too and to help them understand that they can survive the plague of HIV/AIDS. He also knows that many Black gay and bisexual men have been rejected and discarded and has wrapped his arms around as many as he can grab hold of, treating them like family. Sturdevant has two daughters from an early marriage and several grandchildren, but says he feels just as strongly about more than a dozen unrelated "children." He feeds young Black queer people who feel abandoned and need someone they can believe in and who believes in them. Some call him Mr. Ced, others, just Dad.

Despite the persistent anti-LGBT stigma, poverty, and lack of economic and educational opportunity that haunt the South, eroding the health and well-being of its people, Sturdevant feels a complicated, bone-deep, soul tie to the people and the place. When he encourages his "sons" and "daughters" to take care of themselves and others, he is echoing the love and acceptance he received from his own large family. After his years of hiding, when he came out to his mother in his twenties, she told him, "I love you regardless." When his family eventually found out that he was sick, his mother and sister drove up to Memphis, where he was living, along with six carloads of aunts, uncles, nieces, and nephews. They served him plates laden with down-home food that he was too ill to eat and did their best to love him back to health. In the hospital, he finally admitted to his mother he had AIDS. "She told me, 'Boy, you gonna be all right; I got you,'" he recalls, tearing up. In the end, they brought him home. He moved back to Metcalfe, with somebody from the sprawling network of nearly a hundred family members always close by, until he recovered.

As I was working on the final draft of "America's Hidden H.I.V. Epidemic," Sturdevant called to let me know he had resigned from My Brother's Keeper. His new job was manager of the SPOT—Safe Place Over Time—a new initiative, located in a former eyewear shop on the third floor of the Jackson Medical Mall and funded by a pharmaceutical company that produces a dozen HIV medications. He would continue to provide services and support for young gay and bisexual men and transgender women for $8,000 more per year. In his previous job he had been unable to afford Christmas gifts for his children and grandchildren until after the holiday.

When I visited him again in 2020, he had moved back home to the Delta, the poorest area in the poorest state in America. The HIV epidemic in Mississippi remains among the most severe in the country, and the rural Delta counties of Sunflower, Bolivar, and Washington, where Sturdevant is now based, have rates of HIV higher than the state's average. In Greenville, not far from the town where he was raised, Sturdevant was still doing community health work but with more autonomy. He is the director of the nonprofit Community Health-Prevention, Intervention, Education, and Research, also known as CH-PIER, located in a downtown storefront with a few offices, a conference room for support group meetings, a storeroom, and a testing clinic in the back. Washington Avenue, around the corner from his office, looks like the dusty set of a Depression-era film, with its boarded-up buildings, broken windows, peeling paint, and leaves and dirt piled in doorways. Sturdevant spends his days attending health fairs and conferences and conducting seminars at colleges and community centers to raise awareness about HIV/AIDS in the area. He continues to organize monthly support groups for gay and bisexual men and transgender women and has also been trained as a phlebotomist so he can conduct HIV tests and make sure those who end up positive can connect to treatment and care. As we were driving through Greenville, I asked Sturdevant, who has grown his hair into ropy gray locs, making him look like Jesus, Black Jesus, why he moved back home, and he laughed and said, "Sometimes I wonder about that, too." Just then he saw his mother pass us in her dark gray Nissan and called her cell to scold her for driving too fast.

"I think God told me to come back here," he said finally.

Sturdevant functions as a community health worker (CHW), though it's not in his official job title. CHWs are trained health-care providers, chosen because they are trusted members of their communities who act as a bridge between clinical and community settings, between the patient and the provider. They work to improve patient communication and compliance, coordination of care, outreach, prevention, and early diagnoses, particularly in Black and underserved communities. They advocate for patients and offer social support and coaching. Whether they're called patient navigators like Sturdevant or peer recovery coaches like Morgan Anne Wood and Dani Ludwig of the Friendship House in West Virginia, CHWs provide a valuable service where the need is greatest. While CHWs cannot replace quality health-care delivery, they play an important role in increasing access to prevention and treatment services and can help neutralize social and environmental determinants of health that erode the well-being of people and communities. Studies show that CHWs can improve outcomes of chronic illnesses, including diabetes and heart disease, in a wide variety of settings—in urban, rural, and small-town communities as well as in clinics, emergency departments, and veterans' hospitals. They have also been shown to reduce health-care costs. By helping coordinate medical care, offering emotional support, and promoting safe sex and healthy eating, for example, they can avert costly hospitalizations. An article published in February 2020 in the journal *Health Affairs* found that one team of six community health workers serving 330 patients saved the Medicaid program more than $1.4 million a year, for a return of $2.47 for every dollar invested. CHW programs also provide meaningful employment and job creation in communities that need them most.

Still, the United States uses community health workers sparingly, and they remain largely on the fringes of the medical system, underutilized, underpaid, and poorly supported and defined. They lack uniform training or accreditation, their responsibilities and job titles vary, and compensating them fairly has been spotty and ad hoc. In 2010, the Affordable Care Act officially acknowledged CHWs as an important component of the health-care workforce, and several years later a number of states began advancing the CHW infrastructure—professional identity, workforce development, training, and financing—in various ways with legislation. But our country of 331 million employs only about 59,000 CHWs, according to the Bureau of Labor Statistics, a much lower ratio than nations that have made the greatest impact by using CHWs—countries like Ethiopia, which has approximately 42,000 CHWs for a nation less than half the size of ours.

In 2010, I spent two days with Aster Roba, a health extension worker (HEW) in rural Ethiopia. She was one of an army of more than thirty-eight thousand women dispatched by the Ethiopian government to serve as CHWs, beginning in 2004. In Daka Werekelo, where Roba lived and worked, two thousand people reside in a sprawling cluster of mud huts. During my visit, I walked from home to home with Roba as she counseled women about family planning, HIV prevention, hygiene, nutrition, and other healthy practices. We sat in modest homes with dirt floors, children crawling on their mothers like playground equipment, as they listened to Roba with interest and respect and asked her questions mainly about their kids. Roba also dug latrines and distributed mosquito nets and in her clinic inserted birth control implants, administered contraceptive injections, provided prenatal and gynecological care, vaccinated children, and treated diarrhea. On a sweltering morning, she held a community meeting in a field, standing in the middle of a circle of about thirty people in her village to exchange information and voice concerns, on this day primarily about a lack of water for drinking and bathing. Afterward, as we talked in the cramped office she shared with a twenty-year-old colleague, she told me with pride that she had helped women deliver babies in their homes and that she had brought about a dozen children into the world.

HEWs like Roba are an integral part of Ethiopia's health-care system, working to combat a tangle of poverty-fueled health problems, including infant and maternal mortality and child death, in a country with an average of only one physician for every hundred people. In contrast, the United States then had approximately twenty-six doctors for every hundred people. Roba was eligible to become a HEW and go through the yearlong training program because in Ethiopia, where most women are illiterate, she had made it through the tenth grade and could read. She was attracted to the job because of a tragedy in her earlier life: when Roba was fourteen, her mother nearly died in childbirth delivering her tenth child in ten years. In the aftermath, as her mom struggled back to life, a HEW came to her home to talk about family planning, and Roba realized that's what she wanted to do. "I never want someone else to suffer like my mother did," she told me through a translator, surrounded by a rambunctious collection of barefoot children in stained and tattered clothing, giggling and pulling at her skirt.

The HEW program has the added benefit of providing dignified employment for tens of thousands of women, and inspiring young girls who see them as role models: educated, competent, and commanding respect. Since I visited Ethiopia, the HEW program has been evaluated and held up as a model of success, though it still struggles under intractable infrastructure issues like transportation, sanitation, and communication as well as power and water shortages, all of which plague the nation. Ethiopia has made dramatic progress in improving the health outcomes of its population at least partly due to the program. It reduced child deaths by 69 percent, from 205 per 1,000 live births in 1990 to 64 per 1,000 live births in 2013, accomplishing the United Nations Millennium Development Goal 4 three years ahead of schedule. The maternal mortality ratio plummeted from 1,030 maternal deaths per 100,000 live births in 2000 to 401 per 100,000 in 2017. A 2020 report estimated that Ethiopia's army of HEWs saved the lives of more than 50,000 mothers and children between 2008 and 2017. Hygiene and sanitation improvements instituted by HEWs have led to a reduction of major communicable diseases. Additionally, a study that looked at forty-nine peer-reviewed papers published between 2003 and 2018 pointed to health improvements in Ethiopia specifically related to its HEW program. These include significant improvements in maternal and child health, hygiene and sanitation, knowledge and health-care seeking, and a reduction in communicable diseases.

Globally, CHWs—who, depending on the country, are referred to by a variety of names, including lady health workers, *visitadoras,* village health guides, women group leaders—deliver babies, support breast-feeding, administer vaccinations and birth control, manage childhood illnesses, counsel mental health patients, and provide preventive health education on malaria, TB, HIV/AIDS, and sexually transmitted infections. Research from the World Health Organization shows that around the world the services CHWs offer have led to declines in maternal and child mortality rates and decreased incidence of TB and malaria in some of the most disadvantaged nations.

The CHW concept was first conceived in China in the 1950s. At the time, China had an estimated 40,000 physicians serving a population of 540 million people. Most of these doctors worked in large cities, even though 80 percent of the population lived in rural areas. In the 1960s, Chairman Mao, the leader of China's Communist Party, created an army of "barefoot doctors," thousands of young rural men and women who received an intensive three- to six-month course of medical training. When they returned to their villages, they were able to provide basic health care and education. By the 1970s, about a million of these lay professionals served rural areas in China, and the World Health Organization and leaders in other countries gave China's program a hard look as an alternate to expensive, Western-style medical-care models. A compilation of case studies published in 2020 looked at the effectiveness of the many offspring of China's example. The report notes that Bangladesh Rural Advancement Committee employs 43,000 CHWs, who have helped that country reduce under-five mortality and high rates of

TB. In Brazil's Family Health Strategy, 265,000 community health agents offer services such as immunization, family planning, and breast-feeding support, which has helped spark dramatic improvements in a number of national health indicators over the past three decades. Nepal has been a global leader in reducing its under-five mortality, maternal mortality, and fertility rates, with the help of CHWs, who provide reproductive health services, immunize babies, treat childhood illnesses, and offer individual and community health education.

Though we think of this kind of people-driven, low-tech care as a solution only for less wealthy countries, far too many pockets of the United States, inside cities and in large swaths of rural America, are as broken down as or worse off than many of the poorest countries of the world. I was reminded of Aster Roba seven years later, when I met Latona Giwa of the Birthmark Doula Collective. I spent several weeks, off and on, shadowing her in New Orleans in 2017, for my *New York Times* article and recognized in her relationships with her clients the same kind of familiarity, caring, and deep listening I had witnessed in Ethiopia. To be sure, Giwa has more education than a typical CHW. After graduation from Grinnell College in Iowa in 2009, she moved to New Orleans, where she completed an accelerated program in nursing at Louisiana State University. She worked for a year as a labor and delivery nurse and several more as a visiting nurse for Medicaid clients in St. Bernard Parish, where every structure was damaged by Katrina floodwaters. She left nursing to devote herself to doula work and childbirth education, co-founding the nonprofit Birthmark Doula Collective, after observing the lack of services for women in New Orleans who most needed support during pregnancy but couldn't afford it. A 2016 study published in the journal *Birth* shows that women who received doula support had 22 percent lower odds of preterm and cesarean births, and doula care also produced cost savings. The concept of doula care has also spread beyond pregnancy and birth: doulas help women through the process of abortion and assist HIV patients with treatment regimens, and "death doulas" provide support at the end of life.

As I described earlier, Giwa guided Simone Landrum through an emotionally difficult pregnancy following her escape from an abusive relationship, the death of her baby Harmony, and her own near death during childbirth. While Landrum was in labor with her son Kingston in December 2017, Giwa shielded her from appalling treatment by health-care providers in the labor and delivery room. Giwa was the only person during Landrum's tense, touch-and-go delivery who kept her eyes locked on the laboring mother, not the machines in the room. Even after the birth of the baby, Giwa's work was not finished. It was she who drove Landrum and baby Kingston home from the hospital, a tray of homemade lasagna in the back of her car, when there was no one else to do so. Despite her high-risk status, no one had contacted Landrum from her ob-gyn's office about a follow-up appointment after the birth until Giwa asked her about it and made sure she went in. For all of her work, attentiveness, and radical kindness over about five months, Giwa received, as noted, only $600, paid through Birthmark Collective fundraising.

Our nation, even with the most expensive health-care system and arguably the best medical technology in the world, cannot rely only on clinical and technical solutions to dig our way out of the nation's most vexing health issues, which include high rates of infant and maternal mortality and lowered life expectancy compared with other wealthy countries as well as persistent racial disparities in nearly every health outcome. Without a personal connection to offset the largely impersonal nature of the current medical system, spending more and more money on health care will never erase the problems dogging America or close the racial gap. Our country must instead combine the rigorous science and advanced technology we are known for with kindness, care, and support.

In the spring of 2018, Rodneka Shelbia of New Orleans was in the second trimester of a pregnancy with her first baby. At twenty-two weeks, she visited her doctor, alarmed after she noticed she had passed her mucus plug, the protective seal covering the cervical canal in a pregnant woman. She also had back pain, loose bowels, and cramps, which, along with passing the plug, seemed to signal very early labor. Though she insisted to her physician that something was wrong, the doctor ignored her concerns, assuring Rodneka that her pregnancy was normal. She directed her to a pregnancy website and sent her home.

Several days later, the symptoms became more intense, and she began having contractions. Just to be sure, Rodneka looked at the website the doctor had advised her to read, identified the signs of labor, and also noticed that the site listed her previous complaints—passing the mucus plug, back pain, loose bowels, and cramps. Rodneka estimated that she was one day away from twenty-three weeks of pregnancy and understood that babies born earlier than twenty-three weeks have almost no chance of survival. In these cases, clinicians will generally not try to save the baby, but instead let the parents hold the infant immediately after birth until he or she dies, which often happens within minutes. Terrified, Rodneka began praying and talking to her baby girl, begging her not to come, to wait one more day. She did. The following day, with contractions five minutes apart and now bleeding, Rodneka went back to the hospital, only to be sent home again by her doctor, who continued to insist she wasn't in labor. For another excruciating week, Rodneka waited, still bleeding and having contractions. Finally, on April 21, at twenty-four weeks, Iamme was born, weighing one pound six ounces and classified as extremely premature. The tiny infant was immediately whisked into the NICU and remained in the hospital for eight months. Eventually, Rodneka's doctor explained to her that she had suffered placental abruption, which occurs when the placenta partly or completely separates from the wall of the uterus before delivery. The physician admitted that she had missed this diagnosis, but never apologized.

A little over two years later, on September 23, 2020, Rodneka Shelbia told the story of Iamme's birth to a Zoom room of some forty-five physicians, nurses, and other health-care providers and administrators, most from Touro Infirmary, where Rodneka had had her baby, as part of a daylong workshop. I observed, interested to see what had changed in New Orleans since the time I had spent in the city reporting my 2018 *New York Times Magazine* cover story on Black mothers and babies. Louisiana has one of the highest rates of infant mortality in the country, and Black infants are about twice as likely to die before they are old enough to walk. Louisiana is among the states with the highest rates of maternal mortality in the country, and Black mothers die five times more often than white mothers for pregnancy-related reasons, deaths that are nearly always preventable. Touro, a community hospital that serves large numbers of Black women, has elevated rates of severe maternal morbidity—the near death of a pregnant woman—higher than the state average. It is also the hospital where Simone Landrum, the central figure in my article, delivered her stillborn daughter and almost bled to death herself, after her physician ignored her legitimate concerns and signs of dangerously high blood pressure.

Rodneka's presentation was part of an Institute for Healthcare Improvement initiative that brought together doulas from Birthmark, clinicians and administrators from Touro, other Louisiana health-care providers, and Black women from New Orleans. The group works together to redesign maternal care with a focus on improving clinical outcomes and increasing dignity, equity, and safety. The process includes Equity Action Labs and Momentum Labs, gatherings where Black women like Rodneka are active participants in redesigning the way care is delivered. They describe the problems they experienced during delivery and with prenatal and postpartum care with the providers at the facility where they received care, encouraging them to understand and acknowledge the harm they might have unknowingly created.

Projects like these have been developed to address long-standing racial discrimination and bias in medical treatment and care. Despite enough documentation of these phenomena to fill the Library of Congress, the appetite for making significant, systemic change remains halting. Some medical practitioners, health administrators, and governmental officials acknowledge the problem, but in general medicine has been slow to come to terms with it. In 2020, the American Medical Association, the country's largest association of physicians and medical students, finally recognized racism as a public health threat. That announcement came twelve years after the organization, founded before the Civil War, apologized for a history of discrimination against Black doctors.

Solutions have been difficult to come by. Many medical providers, educators, and public health officials find it too overwhelming to confront the problem, wondering—with some justification—how to combat racism that has been embedded in the systems and institutions of America since the birth of the country. Others stubbornly resist discussing the intersection of race, racism, and health care, even as the crisis grows. Carol Hogue, PhD, an Emory University epidemiologist and one of the original authors of the landmark 1992 *New England Journal of Medicine* study on infant mortality in college-educated parents, had warned me about this sort of pushback. When I asked her why she felt the need to include 174 citations from previous work in an article she had published—an epidemiological review of research about the association between racial disparities in preterm birth and interpersonal and institutional racism—her answer was to the point: "No one believes you unless you *really* have evidence behind it. You can't just explain what you know; you have to prove it over and over."

Even those in the field who are more knowledgeable about racial health disparities and social determinants of health often think of the problem in terms of a kind of hierarchy of oppression, insisting that the inequity is less about race and more about class. They generally admit that the elevated rates of poverty in African Americans have their roots in 250 years of slavery, another 100 years of government-sanctioned discrimination and segregation, and continued societal racial bias. But they are slower to grasp that bias in the health-care system extends beyond poor Black Americans and persists even among more advantaged African Americans. So they ask for more—proof, research, data, and documentation. Earlier in this book, I document one of the most important and frequently cited reports on racial bias in medical care, *Unequal Treatment: Confronting Racial and Ethnic Disparities in Health Care.* This gold-standard, book-sized report from 2003 compiles 483 studies that point to unequivocal racial disparities in health-care treatment even after controlling for socioeconomic factors.

This report cuts to the core of the issue, with heartbreaking specificity. One of the studies highlighted looked at medical procedures for patients suffering from diabetes and prostate cancer. It focused only on Medicare patients in order to equalize access to health care in its subjects. Published in *The New England Journal of Medicine,* the 1996 study found that doctors cut off all or part of the legs of their Black patients 3.6 times more frequently than those of their white patients. In 62 percent of amputations, the principal diagnosis was diabetes. The researchers noted that though diabetes is more common in Blacks than whites, the difference in the rates of amputation was not explained by the difference in the prevalence of diabetes. The same study found that bilateral orchiectomy—removal of both testicles—was more than twice as frequent among Black men as among whites. Neither the rates of prostate cancer nor the severity of the cases explained why Black men were more likely to lose their testicles when other less life-altering remedies were available.

This study stopped short of blaming individual health-care providers for what seemed to be racially motivated decisions, and no one believes the doctors and other providers behind the numbers acted with the callousness of an antebellum physician like J. Marion Sims. But someone made these decisions; human beings are responsible for deciding when to cut off another person's leg or his testicles and for making that crushing choice more often in Black patients than white even when other factors seem to be equal.

Physicians and other health-care providers don't pursue medicine to go against their oath to do no harm. They enter the field to help and heal. Still, the majority of physicians are white and bring their individual biases to their work and, without being conscious of it, may have trouble humanizing and empathizing with people who are different from them. Research shows that Black patients benefit from having a Black health-care provider. A 2020 study showed that Black newborn babies in the United States are more likely to survive childbirth if they are cared for by Black doctors, but three times more likely than white babies to die when looked after by white doctors. The mortality rate for white babies was largely unaffected by the doctor's race.

Underrepresentation in the workforce limits Black patients from being treated by physicians who look like them. Aspiring Black doctors often struggle against financial and educational barriers wrought by systemic discrimination. Far too frequently Black students, particularly men, not only face a lack of role models and encouragement but are actively discouraged from pursuing careers in medicine by teachers, guidance counselors, and professors. And even health-care providers of color harbor bias, and in hectic, rushed health-care settings it tends to surface. We are all functioning in a system and society that are riddled with discrimination based on myths and stereotypes that continue to hang on, even centuries later.

Some groups and individuals are pushing for reform. In a widely circulated editorial in the March 19, 2015, edition of *The New England Journal of Medicine,* Mary Bassett, MD, then the New York City commissioner for health, put out a call to action to health-care providers to not shy away from using the word "racism" when they see health inequality. "Health professionals [should] be accountable not only for caring for individual black patients but also for fighting the racism—both institutional and interpersonal—that contributes to poor health in the first place," she wrote. Beginning in 2016, she also instituted mandatory implicit bias training for all the thousands of employees of the New York City Department of Health.

In 2019, California became the first state in the country to respond directly to Dr. Bassett's challenge after clinical improvements in hospital obstetric care failed to make a dent in racial gaps in maternal mortality. In that state, the rate of maternal deaths climbed sharply from 7.7 deaths per 100,000 live births in 1999 to 16.9 in 2006. Similar to U.S. Black women as a whole, African American women in California were roughly four times more likely to die than women in other racial/ethnic groups. In response, the state launched the California Maternal Quality Care Collaborative (CMQCC), a multi-stakeholder organization anchored at Stanford University School of Medicine charged with reducing the deaths of mothers and babies. CMQCC created tool kits—instructions for hospital personnel to make sure that the best protocols and tools were on hand in the case of obstetric emergencies like hemorrhage and dangerously high blood pressure. These evidence-based clinical innovations worked: California saw maternal mortality decline by 55 percent between 2006 and 2013, while the U.S. national maternal mortality rate continued to rise. However, Black women did not benefit, and the racial disparity in maternal mortality between Black and white women in California remained stubbornly in place.

State senator Holly J. Mitchell, a Black woman, and others realized that doctoring their way out of the maternal mortality crisis would never work. So she co-sponsored SB-464, the California Dignity in Pregnancy and Childbirth Act, a bill that, among other things, would require all health-care providers treating pregnant women and delivering babies to undergo implicit bias training to curb the impact of bias on maternal health. California's governor, Gavin Newsom, signed it into law in October 2019, and it went into effect the following year.

Other states have created quality initiatives similar to California's under the umbrella term Perinatal Quality Collaboratives, or PQCs. These are networks of clinical teams, public health leaders, and other partners, including patients and families, that work together to improve pregnancy and infant outcomes. At this point, nearly every state has a PQC at some stage of development. In August 2018, the newly created LaPQC launched the Reducing Maternal Morbidity Initiative to reduce deaths and near deaths of mothers from hemorrhage and hypertension—the leading causes of preventable pregnancy-associated mortality in Black women—by 20 percent in one year. Participation was voluntary, but dozens of hospitals and birthing centers signed on, including Touro as well as Ochsner, where Simone Landrum delivered Kingston. In initial surveys, not a single hospital team mentioned equity, instead focusing on clinical outcomes—reducing hypertension and hemorrhage deaths without the explicit tilt toward racial equity. That sounded like the blind spot the California experiment had encountered: mistakenly assuming that upgrading and standardizing clinical measures would reduce the role that provider bias played and trickle down to narrow the racial disparity in birth outcomes. Instead, the Louisiana team more intentionally embedded antiracism training and community engagement in the work. A group of facilitators conducted workshops to train hospital teams about race, racism, white supremacy, and the role of implicit bias in care and equity. A turning point came in January 2019 during a daylong workshop with 130 physicians, nurses, and hospital administrators at the Cajundome in Lafayette. The organizers brought in LaToshia Rouse, a patient adviser with North Carolina's PQC, to share her birthing experience.

In 2014, LaToshia delivered triplets, born early at twenty-six weeks. Eventually, she returned home, leaving her three tiny babies in the hospital's NICU. Twenty days later, in the middle of the night, LaToshia woke up after feeling something wet in her bed. She made it to the bathroom, turned on the light, and discovered she was hemorrhaging. There was so much blood on the floor that her bathroom looked like a crime scene. She was suffering a postpartum hemorrhage—when a woman experiences heavy blood loss after giving birth—which in the United States is a leading cause of pregnancy-related death and neonatal death, and more common in Black women than other women. Shoving a towel between her legs to soak up the blood, LaToshia called 911, tried not to move, and waited for EMS to arrive. By the time paramedics got to her door, LaToshia was nearly unconscious from blood loss, but through the haze she noticed that the paramedics didn't seem to be acting with urgency. They never checked to see how much blood she had lost, but instead, seeing her having trouble holding her head up, assumed she was using drugs and asked her, repeatedly, what she had "taken" and what she had "done." They then asked LaToshia if she could stand up. When she said no, they persisted, holding her by her arms to help lift her. Weakened by blood loss, she fell. She made it to the hospital for treatment, but still considers this one of the worst days of her life. She is also crystal clear that she would've been treated differently had she been white. "I understand how women die and what happens when someone sees a stereotype, not the person right in front of them," she told the audience in Lafayette. She explained that she shares her personal story in order to illustrate, to really get providers of all stripes to hear, and understand, the pain and trauma that can result when a patient isn't listened to or made a priority.

As a result of the workshop, and hearing LaToshia's and other stories, clinicians and administrators got a clearer picture of the role of racism in patient experiences and also what it looks like when people most impacted by disparities become the drivers of change. Some hospitals in the state, which had been resistant to racial equity training, began voluntarily engaging in it. In the end, after twenty-one months of work to improve hospital practices, including training to recognize and combat implicit racial bias, Louisiana's PQC more than reached its goal: reducing near death from hemorrhage by 39 percent and from hypertension by 22 percent. However, the racial disparities barely budged; most of the improvements benefited white mothers. Still, that group has decided to continue the work, focusing on equipping hospitals to provide safe and racially equitable care.

In general, this kind of training to root out and erase health-care bias in the United States remains patchy, unregulated, and uncoordinated; even the names—implicit bias training, antiracism training, unconscious bias training, diversity training, antibias training, racial-bias training, undoing racism training, equal-opportunity training—lack consistency. It's also unclear, depending on the structure and format, how well it works. Whatever the form, the goal is to fight against the sometimes centuries-old attitudes or images that unconsciously shape understanding, actions, and decisions. Implicit bias, based on views developed throughout life and shaped by societal messages internalized as truths from family, peers, media, and authority figures, results in stereotypes that are lodged in the mind.

The result is overgeneralizing about certain groups that can have devastating effects, especially in medical settings.

Antibias training is far from new; it has existed for decades. Most large companies have some form of diversity training, and federal agencies began requiring staff trainings following the civil rights movement of the 1960s. Still, trainings often lack depth. A single workshop or a one-shot digital training isn't enough to uproot long-standing, deep-rooted biases, and far too often, after the training ends, little has shifted. Many programs use a "good person, bad person" framework rather than looking at discrimination as systemic and institutional. Most acts of racism and bias arise in people with blind spots, not Proud Boys memberships.

The implicit bias training enacted by Mary Bassett at the New York City Health Department took a more holistic approach, examining the impact and existence of racism not only in individuals but throughout the agency, and also considered the broader systemic influences on the organization. The agency used the Undoing Racism model, created by the People's Institute for Survival and Beyond. This New Orleans–based organization has completed twenty thousand trainings and workshops since 1980 and focuses on moving beyond addressing the symptoms of racism to undoing it in order to foster a more just and equitable society. In two-day trainings, participants develop a common definition of racism and an understanding of its different forms: individual, institutional, linguistic, and cultural, the participant's own connection to racism, and its impact on their work. They learn about power and privilege and address how bias and discrimination negatively affect everyone, including white people. Most important, participants build awareness and understanding about ways to begin undoing racism. Health agencies in Boston, Baltimore, and other cities and counties have done similar antibias work.

Following the murder of George Floyd in May 2020 and in the shadow of protests against racism and police violence around the world, the initiative that Rodneka Shelbia and the Birthmark Doulas took part in made the decision to focus explicitly on the role of racism in perinatal outcomes, using restorative justice practices as a framework. More often applied in the criminal justice system, restorative justice puts those who are harmed, wrongdoers, and their affected communities together in search of solutions that promote responsibility, repair, and the rebuilding of relationships while preserving the safety and dignity of everyone involved.

With that lens in mind, during the Zoom workshop in September 2020, after Rodneka Shelbia described her labor and delivery, organizers asked her to tell the providers from Touro Infirmary what restorative justice might look like in the face of so much loss as a result of the treatment she received at their facility. Even as Rodneka made her presentation, Iamme, then two years old, was recovering from yet another surgical procedure, this one on her thyroid, and used a breathing tube to bring oxygen into her lungs. If her doctor had listened to her and made the correct diagnosis, Rodneka might have received an antenatal steroid injection, a standard form of treatment to speed up the development of a preterm baby's lungs. This shot has been shown to lower the risk of breathing problems in infants, and it would have made a difference for Iamme.

As she addressed the Touro providers and administrators, Rodneka struggled to describe what restorative justice might mean for her. Because she had to miss so much work in her daughter's first year of life, Rodneka lost her job, and her marriage broke up as a result of the stress. She considered suing the doctor, but worried that the time, energy, and cost would distract from caring for her child. She was also wary of reliving the trauma, feeling the anger and hurt rush back. Also, if she lost the case, it might feel like a slap in the face, almost as bad as the initial experience. As she spoke, the clinicians and administrators began to better understand what patients like Rodneka may be experiencing on their watch and how they might provide better care in order to prevent avoidable preterm complications.

The process in New Orleans involved more than just confrontation and critique. The organizers also offered an example of the compassionate, equitable care another patient, Quiatta Joseph, received at Touro in order to help frame changes the group would design together. On April 2, 2020, Quiatta, nine weeks pregnant, suffered a miscarriage. By the time she made it to a hospital not far from her home via ambulance, she had lost more than a liter of blood. After being examined by providers in that facility, she was given pain medication and then discharged—still bleeding, barefoot, and wearing only a bloody hospital gown. The follow-up appointment she was given for three days later turned out to be for a day the clinic was closed. Distraught, she called a neighbor to pick her up from the street corner. Her neighbor drove her home, and later, when she began bleeding again, they called Audrey Stewart, a member of the Birthmark Doula Collective and midwifery student who had been involved in the various equity initiatives in the city and state. Stewart phoned ahead to a physician partner at Touro, and a team of Black women residents from Louisiana State University met Quiatta at the door of the emergency room. There, medical personnel explained what the providers had failed to tell her on April 2, that she had miscarried. They gave her a blood transfusion, a dilation and curettage procedure, or D&C, and antibiotics. They even allowed her to call her mother to say a prayer for the lost infant. As Quiatta told her story during the workshop, she wept at the painful memory but also with gratitude.

An important outcome of all of this effort was that Touro opened an obstetric emergency department, hiring four physicians so that patients arriving with obstetric emergencies are seen immediately by an ob-gyn instead of first being evaluated by a regular ER doctor. This process might have saved the life of Simone Landrum's stillborn daughter.

The problems with clinicians that the Louisiana initiatives and others are attempting to address start early, in medical school. Even as the country grows more diverse, only 12 percent of medical school graduates were Black, Latinx, or Native American as of the 2018–2019 academic year. Beginning in the eighteenth century, U.S.

medical schools routinely taught theories that created and perpetu-
ated racial inferiority, mythology, and stereotypes. The practice bled
into modern times as medical schools continued to teach race as a
risk factor for a number of diseases and to use faulty algorithms with
built-in race corrections for diagnosis and treatment across various
fields of medicine. The much-cited 2016 University of Virginia study
of medical students and residents and their skewed perceptions of
pain in Black versus white patients and their false assumptions about
Black bodies made it clear that racial stereotypes and unconscious
bias continue to poison health-care providers while they are in training and have the power to corrupt their eventual medical decision
making.

But medical education is shifting, and growing numbers of medical schools across the country acknowledge the problem of racial bias
in medicine and are addressing implicit or unconscious bias before it
infects doctors-to-be. Far too often, though, it is not medical school
administrators who are spurring action but the students themselves
even as they balance the pressing demands of schoolwork. I was interested to see if there had been any changes in the medical schools
in New Orleans. There, students train at the hospitals where Simone
Landrum received subpar treatment and care. I learned that a group
of students at Louisiana State University School of Medicine had
taken a close look at how racial equity was covered in their curriculum and found it lacking. In 2017 they created the Critical Consciousness in Medicine project, which supplements their normal
medical school curriculum. Madeleine DeGrange, one of four medical student leaders in the 2020–2021 school year, conducts two-hour
sessions every month that examine implicit bias, institutional racism, health disparities, and other topics. Eventually, she would like
to practice ob-gyn, but for now she is a full-time student while also
functioning as a professor of sorts, gathering materials, recruiting
speakers, and delivering monthly TED-like talks to the mostly white
students in the class below hers.

DeGrange, who is Black, says that an experience working as a
medical scribe set her on a path not just to acquire medical educa-

tion but to help transform it. In 2018, after she graduated from the University of Miami with a degree in biology, she had a year to kill before she started medical school at LSU. During that gap year, she took a job as a medical scribe at Ochsner Medical Center in her hometown—the hospital where Simone Landrum had Kingston. This was an ideal interim job for DeGrange, the daughter of an anesthesiologist father and psychologist mother. She was responsible for taking notes for physicians during interviews with patients in the ER and writing up the encounters on medical charts. She hoped this experience would prepare her for her eventual role as a doctor herself and teach her how to listen deeply to patients in order to improve their care and treatment. But what she observed was the opposite; she was shocked by how little some of the ER physicians, mainly white, actually listened to their patients, primarily people of color. Instead, the doctors in the rushed emergency room environment cut off patients mid-sentence, hurrying them along and talking over them, denying them the time or space to tell their stories. The doctors made assumptions about the patients, not allowing them to speak for themselves or be proactive in their treatment decisions. DeGrange saw the frustration and fear in the faces of those patients, and she was reminded of her experience as a Katrina survivor.

In August 2005, when the hurricane hit New Orleans and destroyed her home and everything inside it, Madeleine DeGrange was just ten years old. Her family—her parents and two brothers—evacuated, first to Houston for two months, then to Houma, a town about an hour southwest of New Orleans, before they were eventually able to return home. That experience of fear, grief, loss, and displacement is part of the DeGrange family lore. Their story defines them and is integral to who they are. As Madeleine grew into adulthood, she understood that remembering the experience and sharing it was part of the healing for all of those who survived the hurricane. Similarly, she understood that for patients, telling their stories and being heard is part of the healing, and hearing them should be part of the job of physicians and other health-care providers. For providers, listening to patients encourages sound treatment and care decisions. Part of her goal now is to make sure that implicit bias and unconscious racial discrimination aren't preventing her classmates and her from listening to and fairly treating patients who may be different from them.

On a national level, students at more than seventy U.S. medical schools have come together to form White Coats for Black Lives with the goal of eliminating racial bias in medicine and pushing medical schools to teach more about racial justice. They believe that the medical schools they attend and their affiliated hospitals where they first practice have failed to promote racial equity. Moved to action by the deaths of Eric Garner and Michael Brown and inspired by the Black Lives Matter movement, in 2014 students at the University of California, San Francisco School of Medicine, the Icahn School of Medicine at Mount Sinai, and the Perelman School of Medicine at the University of Pennsylvania put out a call, mainly through social media, for their peers of all races to stand in solidarity with communities protesting against racism and police brutality. On December 10, 2014, International Human Rights Day, some three thousand students at more than eighty medical schools across the country participated in a national die-in, publicly stating that health professionals must confront police violence and institutionalized racism. Under the hashtag #whitecoats4blacklives, their actions trended on social media and were covered by traditional media. In 2019, the group published its first Racial Justice Report Card to evaluate medical colleges on the basis of fourteen metrics, such as student and faculty diversity, racial integration of clinical care sites, treatment of workers, and research protocols that protect people of color from abusive practices. With these report cards, they hope to encourage academic medical centers to take seriously their responsibility to fight racism in the field.

On the West Coast, in 2020, a group of students in a joint MD/ MPH program at the UCSF School of Medicine and Berkeley School of Public Health launched the Institute for Healing and Justice in Medicine. It had its roots in a class four students took in 2018 with Osagie K. Obasogie, PhD, an expert in bioethics who specializes in examining the hidden ways racial thinking has crept into medicine and science. As they learned more from their professor about the history of bias in medicine and the ways racism creates health disparities, they began to question the ways race was "biologized" in their textbooks and classes. Racial health disparities, they believe, are often wrongly attributed to biology and physiology of racial groups rather than to forms of oppression that create inequality. They also worried that in clinical practice they were mentored by clinicians who blindly follow guidelines that instruct them to prescribe based on race rather than overall effectiveness, even though the guidelines are built on a history of racism in medicine and health care. In response, the multiracial student group, all women, wrote "Towards the Abolition of Biological Race in Medicine: Transforming Clinical Education, Research, and Practice," an exhaustive, evidence-based, peer-reviewed manifesto that argues that discrimination must be abolished in medicine and clinical research, education, and practice. They launched the report online in May 2020, and more than seven thousand people, primarily other med students, attended the national unveiling, and thousands more have viewed it since.

Beyond the individual decision making that may be tainted by implicit bias in health-care providers, student groups and others have focused specifically on the calculations and algorithms used to help physicians make medical decisions. In theory, the science behind medicine should be objective, rational, and evidence based, but like the race correction in measuring lung function, advanced centuries ago by the infamous Dr. Samuel Cartwright and still present in medical education and practice, these calculations can be blemished by racism. In August 2020, a study published in *The New England Journal of Medicine* found that algorithms used by hospitals and clinicians to guide medical decisions for tens of millions of Americans are contaminated by implicit racism and can result in Black people receiving inferior care. And students are still learning these flawed concepts in medical school.

The Institute for Healing and Justice in Medicine and other groups and individuals have been advocating for medical providers to abandon the race correction embedded in a common test for kidney function and for medical schools to stop teaching it. To determine kidney health, clinicians first measure factors such as the level of creatinine, a by-product of muscle breakdown, in the blood. Poorly functioning kidneys have a more difficult time filtering out creatinine, and a high level suggests that the renal system is not performing well. Physicians use an equation to combine this information into an eGFR score. In a Black patient, the eGFR is multiplied by a factor of 1.21, which makes kidney function look artificially better in Black patients even in the face of serious kidney problems. Underlying this race correction is the false assumption that Black people have more muscle mass than other individuals and thus higher levels of creatinine. Though I would never be referred to as muscular, while I was finishing this book, my own eGFR test came back with two options: one score if I were white, and a race-corrected option for me, a Black patient. These outmoded practices can have real consequences: African Americans suffer from kidney failure at a rate three times higher than whites and make up 35 percent of all patients receiving dialysis for kidney failure; the faulty test means that Black people must meet higher eGFR thresholds of kidney function in order to be diagnosed with kidney disease compared with individuals of other racial groups.

In 2020, Naomi Nkinsi, one of five Black students in her class at the University of Washington School of Medicine in Seattle, succeeded in getting her college to stop teaching this incorrect calculation. During a lecture, she was taught that race plays a role in kidney function with no further explanation. Concerned, she asked her professor, "What is the physiological pathway that links melanin to kidney function? How do you identify a patient as Black? What happens if the patient is mixed race or doesn't look Black to the physician, but has Black ancestry?" And the only response she received was that Black people have more muscle mass. Period.

Angered and alarmed, she partnered with her college's Anti-racism Action Committee and rallied other students and eventually some faculty members to force the school to stop teaching the race correction. Her coalition was able to show that there is no evidence of physiological difference in kidney function between Black patients and others. In May 2020, her school officially made the change. Other students at medical schools across the country have pressed their colleges to follow suit.

This section is supposed to be about hope, and I am excited by the energy and activism of the new generation of medical students, inspired by the commitment and kindness of community health workers—no matter what they are called—and hopeful that antiracism training can root out bias in individual providers. But sometimes hope gets slapped with a hard dose of reality: in September 2019, Stanley Goldfarb, MD, former associate dean of curriculum at the University of Pennsylvania's Perelman School of Medicine, published an essay in *The Wall Street Journal*, "Take Two Aspirin and Call Me by My Pronouns."

"At 'woke' medical schools, curricula are increasingly focused on social justice rather than treating illness," he wrote, arguing for a rigorous curriculum that prepares students for today's rapidly advancing medical science, rather than turning them into advocates for social and political issues. Three days later, the *Journal*'s op-ed page followed up with a piece cheerleading Dr. Goldfarb's beliefs and condemning his critics. In April 2020, during the height of the COVID-19 pandemic, the *Journal* published another essay by Dr. Goldfarb in which he insisted that medical school curricula had ignored public health and disaster preparedness in favor of social issues. During an interview in 2021, Dr. Goldfarb argued with me that focus on racial disparities in maternal mortality was misguided and flawed.

In March 2021, during a podcast about structural racism in medicine, the deputy editor of the prestigious *Journal of the American Medical Association* stated, "Structural racism is an unfortunate term. Personally, I think taking racism out of the conversation will help. Many people like myself are offended by the implication that we are somehow racist." A tweet about the podcast from *JAMA*'s Twitter account followed: "No physician is racist, so how can there be structural racism in health care?" Though the tweet and podcast have been deleted and the deputy editor and the editor in chief—both white male physicians—resigned, I was reminded of something one of my role models, the activist and author Audre Lorde, said to me. I asked her, before she passed away in 1992, if she thought racism in our country was dying out. She suggested that I was being overly optimistic and warned me that when something dies, it doesn't just fade away; it fights to the death, desperately clinging to life, and goes out ugly. Bias and discrimination in medicine—and resistance to believing that they are real—may be receding, but they seem to be going out ugly.

AFTERWORD

At the end of January 2020, as I was writing the last third of this book, I was invited to moderate a panel discussion at the Robert Wood Johnson Foundation's Sharing Knowledge health conference. In February, I joined the two panelists, Joia Crear-Perry and Susan Beane, both Black women physicians, on a planning call. Right away, Joia, a friend and the outspoken, activist founder of an organization called National Birth Equity, wondered why our panel had the dry-as-dust title "Healthcare Bias and Discrimination: Impacts on Maternal and Child Health." "Why are we saying bias and discrimination?" she asked. "Why not just call it what it is—racism?" I remember that my stomach lurched. We would not be the first to say it out loud; others had called out racism in health care, most memorably, as mentioned previously, Dr. Mary Bassett, the former New York City health commissioner, in her 2015 *New England Journal of Medicine* essay, "#BlackLivesMatter—a Challenge to the Medical and Public Health Communities." Still, it seemed aggressive, even hostile, to stake that claim in a room of mainly white health-care providers and public health professionals. It felt as if we were accusing these generally well-meaning people of being racist. The three of us knew that the underlying problem was racism, and I probably felt it most strongly at that moment, because I was in the middle of the deepest dive of my career, cataloging the reasons behind four hundred years of racial health disparities for this book. But I felt uncomfortable owning it. After much back-and-forth,

Joia, bless her, convinced us that we should name the culprit behind the damage to Black bodies explicitly, and we settled on calling the panel "Racism and Bias in Healthcare and Its Impact on Maternal and Child Health."

That conference ended up being the last big gathering I attended before the COVID pandemic hit. When I returned home to Brooklyn on March 6, about a dozen New Yorkers had been diagnosed with the virus. By the end of the month, New York City would be ground zero, with hospitals overwhelmed with patients, ventilators in short supply, refrigerated trucks parked around the city full of bodies waiting to be buried, and my social media pages inundated with fear, sickness, and death.

Now in lockdown, I was spending much more time on my computer. As coronavirus cases in the United States swelled, politicians, physicians, and health experts were warning the public to stay inside and starting to recommend wearing masks, even as the president and his administration were downplaying the danger. Many experts and leaders referred to the coronavirus as a great equalizer, insisting that the disease didn't discriminate. They crafted this broad-based public health message to get all Americans to fall in line with safety rules. But I also started noticing a different conversation. In other circles, talk of the intersection of race and COVID had begun to simmer. My friend the writer Hilary Beard held the first in a series of Facebook live discussions in late March aimed at people of color. She was joined by Phill Wilson, the leading voice of the Black AIDS movement, and Camara Jones, MD, a former president of the American Public Health Association (APHA), a physician, and an expert in racial health inequality. These talks, called "Something Inside: Tools to Thrive, We Gonna Be Alright," were intended to help Black, brown, and other people with marginalized identities protect themselves during the pandemic. Hilary hosted them, she explained, because "mainstream media and public health institutions focus exclusively on white America and leave us to fend for ourselves." The first episode detailed how viruses spread and why Black Americans were at elevated risk for COVID. It received almost three thousand views.

I was also reading notes and comments posted by some of the nearly four thousand members of the Spirit of 1848 Listserv, a caucus of the APHA. Nancy Krieger, PhD, a professor of social epidemiology at the Harvard T. H. Chan School of Public Health, had launched this platform in 1994 to bring together people concerned about social inequalities in health. The inside-baseball name of the group refers to notable events in public health that occurred around that year in response to a worldwide cholera epidemic. One of the goals of the group and its Listserv was to make connections to overcome the isolation that these progressive-minded public health experts felt as they strategized to eliminate social inequity in health. As COVID increased throughout March, that platform caught fire, flooded with animated discussions about the ways people of color were disproportionately affected by this fast-moving disease. Still, it was early days: As Krieger saw a crisis rising, she tried to get the word out in academic and scientific circles by publishing papers predicting a racial divide in COVID outcomes. They were turned down by all of the major medical journals.

At the end of March, Aletha Maybank, MD, a former colleague of Dr. Bassett's at the New York City Health Department and now chief health equity officer and vice president of the American Medical Association, reached out to me. She wanted help getting an op-ed published in *The New York Times* imploring laboratories, health institutions, state and local health departments, and the Department of Health and Human Services to collect and publish coronavirus race and ethnicity statistics. At the time, the only racial data was piecemeal, released by state and city governments. But the picture was becoming clear: In Milwaukee County, Blacks represented only one-quarter of the population but 45 percent of coronavirus cases and 70 percent of COVID-related deaths. And in Chicago, Blacks made up half of all cases and almost three-fourths of deaths, even though the city is 32 percent Black. The lack of coordinated release of racial data was fanning conspiracy theories on the ground; a fallacious idea had begun to circulate on social media that Black people were immune to the coronavirus, supposedly because melanin protected against it. This magical thinking became so rampant that on March 17, the day after announcing that he had tested positive for the disease, the actor Idris Elba posted a Twitter live video that denounced the rumors. "There are so many stupid, ridiculous conspiracy theories about Black people not being able to get it," he said. "That's dumb, stupid."

Like Dr. Maybank, a small but influential group of politicians, medical organizations, and advocacy groups were also agitating, mostly behind the scenes, for more statistics based on race. On March 27, Senators Kamala Harris, Elizabeth Warren, and Cory Booker and Representatives Ayanna Pressley and Robin Kelly, all Democrats, sent a letter to Alex Azar, secretary of the Department of Health and Human Services, urging the agency to reveal racial data on testing and treatment for the virus. Shortly after, the American Medical Association, the American Academy of Pediatrics, the National Medical Association, and other groups sent a similar letter, pressing for coronavirus data by race. The NAACP, Dr. Crear-Perry, and other individuals and organizations separately wrote to Surgeon General Jerome Adams and the CDC chief, Robert Redfield, around the same time, adding a warning that data showing disproportionate COVID numbers might lead to racially motivated stereotyping and harassment. That would prove ominously prescient.

I listened and read and knew in my gut that the concerns were, sadly, justified. Years of reporting on HIV/AIDS in African Americans helped frame my understanding. Epidemics, as COVID was shaping up to be, are not equalizers; instead, they strike at the fissures of inequality. They do discriminate: the spread of disease exposes preexisting patterns of marginalization, bias, and inequality.

On the last day of March, I sent a note to Jessica Lustig, my editor at *The New York Times Magazine,* to give her a heads-up about the discussions about race and COVID that I was hearing. At the time, few news outlets had covered the local data or written about the racial disparities that were beginning to emerge. I explained to Jessica that Hilary Beard and Camara Jones had tried to place an op-ed about the topic in the *Times* and a number of other media outlets but were turned down. Their piece ran in a lesser-known publication targeted to progressive people of color. I warned Jessica that they and others who took part in their Facebook live gatherings mentioned a few times that "mainstream media doesn't care about this." I suggested that she commission an essay by Nancy Krieger, Mary Bassett, Camara Jones, or David Williams of Harvard about the topic and that I'd consult. She responded right away and asked for a more fleshed-out pitch, not for an essay, but for a story I would report and write that answered the questions, why is this disease so devastating to Black Americans, and what set the stage for the negative health outcomes?

By the end of the week, I had an assignment, and a very short deadline: not the usual months and months; because the disease was evolving so quickly, the article would be due in just three weeks. As is my style, I set out to figure out whose story to share to add a human face to the larger themes. By then Louisiana, where I had spent so much time reporting on maternal and infant mortality, had become the first state to release data by race, and the numbers showed a vastly unequal distribution in deaths. While African Americans were 32 percent of the population, they made up 70 percent of the dead. Both Joia Crear-Perry and Audrey Stewart of the Birthmark Doula Collective asked if I knew what was going on with the Zulu Social Aid and Pleasure Club. Founded in 1909, the club is a brotherhood of some eight hundred men, nearly all of them Black, known for community service, civic engagement, celebrating Black pride and excellence, and throwing massive events during Mardi Gras. I looked at the group's Facebook page and saw the Zulu's chaplain had posted a series of messages asking for prayers for several members who were ill followed by brown praying hands emojis. As I continued scrolling, he also announced that several others "had gotten their wings," including Brother Cornell Charles. Eventually, I saw an announcement for the virtual funeral of Mr. Charles, whom everyone called

Dickey, a nickname from childhood. On April 3, along with hundreds of others, I watched his service at Zion Travelers First Baptist Church and learned about the life of this kind, decent husband, father, and community leader who had died of COVID at age fifty-one. During New Orleans's carnival season, he had been a hardworking, behind-the-scenes player for joyful Zulu celebrations, including the Mardi Gras parade. That year, the six weeks of festivities brought more than a million visitors from around the world streaming into the warm, welcoming city to celebrate face-to-face, elbow to elbow with local residents in a succession of street parties and parades.

Dickey had attended almost every one of the Zulu club's carnival season activities, a series of meticulously planned and eagerly awaited ceremonies, balls, festivals, and other events, beginning in January. On February 25, the final day of carnival season, he rose early, put on the Zulu club's signature uniform, a honey-yellow jacket, black sash, and armband that meant he was part of the group's parade organizing committee, and spent the next ten hours fussing over the logistics of the exuberant, chaotic Krewe of Zulu parade. When the Zulus rolled onto Jackson Avenue to kick off Mardi Gras festivities, for Black New Orleans the party started. Tens of thousands of people lined the four-and-a-half-mile route, reveling in the animated succession of jazz musicians, high-stepping HBCU marching bands, and loose-limbed dancing characters dressed in Zulu costumes, complete with grass skirts and blackface makeup, a satirical spit in the eye to the past when Mardi Gras was put on by clubs of white men who barred Black people (and women) from taking part in the festivities. As revelers stood shoulder to shoulder and several feet deep on that late February day, hoping to catch a painted coconut, the "throw" that is the Zulu parade's signature and coveted prize, no one had any idea that this joyous gathering would turn out to be a coronavirus hothouse.

About ten days after the Krewe of Zulu parade, Dickey told his wife he wasn't feeling well. A courier for GE Healthcare, Dickey rose most days around 2:00 a.m. to deliver medical supplies to hospitals and clinics on the morning graveyard route. His second shift—as a supervisor at the New Orleans Recreation Development Commission and baseball, football, and girls' basketball coach at Lusher Charter School—left him little time for rest. Layering on a month-and-a-half whirlwind of Zulu carnival activities was taxing for Dickey, though he rarely let on. He was an easygoing, humble mountain of a man and father of two daughters. At six feet and 260 pounds he carried his weight well, and his middle-age body hadn't shifted far from his days as a three-sport high school athlete. But he also had a number of health conditions, including hypertension, diabetes, and kidney disease, that he mostly managed quietly. His wife, Nicole, who worked as a medical administrator, kept a watchful eye on him, but also says he worked hard to care for himself. He was very good about taking three different blood pressure medications, two kinds of insulin, and another medication for his kidneys. Nicole said she didn't have to fight him, never had to fuss.

Burnell Scales, Nicole's father and also a Zulu member, knew something was wrong Sunday, March 8, when he showed up at the Charleses' expecting to see his son-in-law stirring a giant pot of gumbo or red beans or heaping shrimp, crawfish, and crabs onto plates for the parade of friends, family, and Zulu members who came by every week after church for an open-door hangout and to watch Saints games during football season. When he found out Dickey wasn't in the kitchen as usual but in bed, he started to worry.

On March 12, Dickey told Nicole he still didn't feel well, and his fever had been up and down, spiking as high as 102. His wife stayed close to him, administering fluids and Tylenol, assuming he had the flu. That day she insisted he go to urgent care, where he was tested for the flu. When he didn't have it, he was sent home with no mention of COVID. Nicole's anxiety kicked in the following day when Dickey lost his appetite. He loved food, and even if he was sick, he would eat. She also worried that he needed to eat something because he couldn't take medications to control his blood pressure, diabetes, and kidney problems on an empty stomach. That Friday Nicole told him, "Baby, if you aren't feeling good tomorrow, we're going to the hospital."

On Saturday, March 14, when her husband told her he felt faint, Nicole dragged him to the emergency room at Ochsner Medical Center. The hospital was on lockdown as a result of the growing number of coronavirus cases that had begun to grip the city. That day the Louisiana Department of Health reported 103 cases of the virus, 75 of them in Orleans Parish, and the first death. In the ER, Dickey was again tested for the flu, and again he didn't have it. No one suggested a COVID test, though doctors and other providers were all wearing protective gear. By that evening, he was lying in a hospital bed, attached to fluids. He never left.

On Sunday, March 15, Dickey's oxygen levels had become unstable, fever spiking and breaking, but still none of the health-care providers mentioned COVID or suggested a test. Late that evening, a chest X-ray showed pneumonia, his lungs flooded with fluid. Nicole, who had been sleeping on a reclining chair in the room next to her husband, said one of the doctors told her it was time for an honest conversation. "They said, 'Your husband is much sicker than he looks,'" she remembers. "'His lungs will not be functioning much longer. We need to vent him.'" That was also the day her husband was finally tested for COVID-19.

Nicole was able to stay with her husband for the next three days, locked to his side. Attached to the ventilator, but unable to speak, he looked surprisingly peaceful and even vital. She kept up a vigil of prayer, whispering, "I love you," over and over. She played gospel music on Pandora on her phone, taking comfort in the song "The Blood Still Works." "It's still healing," she sang to him. "There is power in the blood of Jesus, the blood still works." She also had Dickey's phone with her and did her best to field an avalanche of calls from worried family and Zulu brothers. She told them to please keep Dickey in prayer.

On Wednesday, March 18, while Nicole was in the midst of praying, Dickey opened his eyes. "I said to him, 'Baby, you opened your eyes for me. I love you so much,'" and that was the last time she saw his eyes open. On Thursday, March 19, hospital administrators told Nicole she could no longer visit her husband because of a shortage of personal protective equipment. That day, Louisiana's caseload had increased to 392 cases from 280 the day before. At a news conference, the governor of Louisiana announced that the state's health-care system could be overwhelmed in seven to ten days on the current trajectory.

On Tuesday, March 24, a team of hospital medical providers called Nicole. Dickey's blood pressure had dropped, and his kidneys had failed. They told her he wasn't going to make it and he would be removed from the vent. After inquiring about their exposure to coronavirus, administrators allowed Nicole and Dickey's adult daughters, Bethaney and Le'Treion, to come to his room. Wearing gowns, gloves, and masks, they prayed over his body and said good-bye. At 1:33, when Dickey took his last breath, Nicole, his wife of thirty years, was alone by his side. She left her husband in God's hands and asked Him to let Dickey rest, let him go in peace. The following day, as Nicole faced down staggering grief, she received a call that Dickey's COVID test had come back positive.

Nicole shared her story of love and loss with me at the beginning of April, not long after her husband's funeral. The Zulu Social Aid and Pleasure Club had its origins at the intersection of discrimination and death. After emancipation, formerly enslaved Africans, financially crippled in the face of continued Jim Crow oppression, struggled to bury their dead. So they pooled their money by forming social aid clubs to provide dignified, respectful funerals. But COVID had broken the Zulu club's long-standing tradition of sending off fallen brothers with second-line funerals, the New Orleans tradition of celebrating lives of those who have died with a spirited procession of pageantry, jazz, and dance. On April 3, fewer than a dozen people came together at Zion Travelers First Baptist Church to say goodbye to Dickey Charles. They sat scattered throughout the pews in the chapel in observance of the guidelines the City of New Orleans had put into place on March 16, which restricted gatherings. But Nicole and her family managed to livestream the service, and another six hundred people watched from home.

As I continued my reporting, Dr. Maybank's op-ed ran in the

Times on April 7, and the next day the CDC released the first chunk of statistics on COVID and race. The limited data set, of 1,482 coronavirus patients hospitalized in fourteen states, indicated that despite making up 18 percent of those studied, Black people accounted for a third of all severe cases. Data from the Louisiana Department of Health showed that the neighborhoods in Orleans Parish with the largest numbers of Black residents had been hit hardest.

As I traced a trail of blame for the deaths among the Zulus, I examined the state of the pandemic and the response of the White House at the time Dickey and his brothers were unwittingly attending what we would later understand to be "super-spreader" events. On Friday, February 21, the Charles family joined some twenty thousand people packed into the New Orleans Ernest N. Morial Convention Center, the only venue large enough to hold the crowd that came to eat and drink and dance—floor-length ball gowns and tuxedos required—and witness the crowning of the Zulu king and queen of Mardi Gras. On the Sunday after the ball, President Trump set the tone for the country, the state of Louisiana, and the city of New Orleans when he said at a press conference, "The coronavirus is very much under control in the USA." On Monday, February 24, when an estimated 200,000 people spent the day at the Zulu-hosted Lundi Gras, enjoying a smorgasbord of New Orleans food and music on three stages at Woldenberg Park along the Mississippi River, the president reiterated on Twitter that the disease was "under control." The next day, an official from the Centers for Disease Control issued a far bleaker warning than any before about the spread of the virus in the United States, noting that disruptions to life could be severe. Yet the president was still downplaying the risk. He continued to reassure the country that the number of confirmed cases "within a couple of days is going to be down close to zero." On March 9, the day Louisiana confirmed its first case of COVID-19 and as Dickey got sicker and sicker, Trump compared the virus to the flu on Twitter and also tweeted, "The Fake News Media and their partner, the Democrat Party is doing everything within its semi-considerable power (it used to be greater) to inflame the

CoronaVirus situation, far beyond what the facts would warrant." By the time my story closed on April 24, I was livid. The day before, at a White House press briefing, President Trump erroneously suggested that injecting the human body with a disinfectant like bleach or rubbing alcohol could combat the virus, in his words, "knocking it out in a minute." By then, at least thirty members of the Zulu club had been diagnosed with COVID-19. Eight had died or would soon be dead.

My story ran in the *Times* magazine on Sunday, May 3, with the cover line "Who Lives? Who Dies?" in black letters on a stark white background. Along with Dickey Charles's story and the fate of the Zulu club, the piece looked at the ways coronavirus had disproportionately affected Black people, examining the history of racial health disparities in America and emphasizing the cruel realities that had been brought into sharper focus during the pandemic: higher rates of many diseases, in this new context known as underlying conditions; discrimination in medical care; and the social determinants of health, including pollution, that make Black communities less healthful.

Three weeks after the article appeared, as COVID-19 had turned from epidemic to pandemic proportions, a Black man named George Floyd was arrested for a minor offense in Minneapolis and was subsequently murdered by a white police officer. A viral cell-phone video of Floyd's death set off protests across the United States. The glaring injustice of his murder forced a conversation about institutional racism and racial justice to the surface, and his dying words, "I can't breathe," became a rallying cry, galvanizing a movement. In a horrifying intersection between Floyd's death and COVID-19's disproportionate blow on the Black community, autopsy results in June showed that George Floyd had COVID when he was killed.

After I returned to working on this book, I could see that I was living through its latest chapter. When a robust set of data about race and COVID appeared, this longtime health disparity was on full display. African Americans were more likely to come into contact with the virus and were hospitalized at much higher rates than white people, and the Black death rate was twice as high as the white rate. This pileup of deaths led to an even greater racial disparity in life expectancy: In the aftermath of COVID, life expectancy had fallen for everyone, but Blacks lived an average of 2.7 years less, compared with 0.8 for whites, according to CDC data about the first half of 2020 released in 2021. The life expectancy gap between Black and white Americans, which had been decreasing, had expanded to 6 years, the widest racial disparity since 1998.

What's more, conditions like diabetes, stroke, and heart disease that strike Black Americans at younger ages led to Black people like Dickey Charles dying young from this new virus. An analysis of CDC data showed that in every age category, Black people were dying from COVID at roughly the same rate as white people more than a decade older. Among those aged forty-five to fifty-four, Black death rates were at least six times higher than for whites.

When I saw these numbers pointing to worse COVID outcomes for Black people at younger ages, I immediately thought of Arline Geronimus's weathering theory. When I reached out to her, she told me she wasn't surprised by what we were seeing. If Black people's bodies have been prematurely aged by the chronic stress of battling back racism in America, leading to the very underlying health conditions that make COVID more deadly, then weathering would make the virus more deadly.

The early response to the statistics from politicians and even some scientists, however, was more in line with the stale idea that something intrinsic to blackness was leading to the higher hospitalization and death rates among African Americans. The notion that Black bodies are genetically inferior was born centuries ago and advanced by doctors and scientists as a way to justify slavery, as we have seen. In an April radio interview, Louisiana's senator Bill Cassidy, a physician by training, insisted without evidence that genetic reasons put African Americans at risk of diabetes and triggered serious coronavirus complications. An article in *The Lancet* attributed racial disparities in COVID-19 deaths partially to "genetic make-up." Dr. Anthony Fauci, the country's leading expert on infectious disease, shot down that false belief in July, explaining during an interview, "It's not genetic." His background as an HIV/AIDS researcher and his understanding that viruses, including both COVID and HIV, disproportionately impact Black and other marginalized communities, informed his views.

Prominent physicians also began to spout a wounding trope to explain the underlying conditions that worsened COVID-19 outcomes: that Black people were doing something wrong—being careless, ignorant, and irresponsible. Surgeon General Jerome Adams, who is Black himself, chimed in early, implying that individual behavior was leading to higher deaths from COVID-19 among African Americans. At a White House press briefing on April 10, he told "communities of color . . . to step up and help stop the spread so that we can protect those who are most vulnerable." Dr. Adams added that African Americans and Latinos should "avoid alcohol, tobacco, and drugs." He went on, "We need you to do this, if not for yourself, then for your *abuela*. Do it for your granddaddy. Do it for your big mama. Do it for your pop-pop." Dr. Adams walked back his comments, but they stung, especially coming from a Black physician who had spoken openly of his own struggles with pre-diabetes, hypertension, and asthma.

And just as some of the experts had warned, after cities with sizable populations of Black people began to report large numbers of COVID-19 infections at the beginning of April, and statistics showed disproportionate death rates for African Americans, a counternarrative began to arise: the national, state, and local shutdowns were too draconian; the coronavirus pandemic was not as much of a threat—at least not to *all* Americans—as had been argued. Protesters, encouraged by the Trump administration, insisted that others—read: Black and brown people—should take "personal responsibility" in order to turn around the COVID numbers and open up the economy. A smattering of demonstrations broke out the week of April 13, as protesters gathered in a handful of states to push back against stay-at-home orders.

Antiscience rhetoric, including the false idea that wearing a mask does not stop the spread of the virus, trickled down from the White House and into the streets. President Trump and members of his administration downplayed the dangers posed by the coronavirus and undermined efforts to contain it by belittling masks and social-distancing rules, and eventually urging his supporters to protest state lockdown rules put in place to keep residents safe during the pandemic. I watched a video of a "You Can't Close America" rally in Austin, Texas, on April 18, where hundreds of demonstrators, nearly all white, defied social-distancing guidelines by gathering on the steps of the capitol. The protesters—many without masks and out-fitted with Trump hats and flags—shouted, "Let us work" and "Fire Fauci." A woman wearing a "Keep America Great" cap waved a sign reading, "My Life, My Death, My Choice, Personal Responsibility," and another protester held a hand-drawn poster that read, "My Life! Not Yours!"

Saner, more knowledgeable, and more experienced voices rejected the belief that a lack of personal responsibility led to higher rates of coronavirus cases in areas where Black people and other people of color lived. Instead, they pointed to racial segregation, a by-product of systemic racism, as the problem. As discussed in chapter 5 of this book, Black people are more likely than whites to live in communi-ties with high rates of poverty, where physical and social structures are crumbling, where opportunity is low and unemployment high. Even educated, affluent Black people live in poorer neighborhoods, on average, than white people with working-class incomes.

The conditions in the social and physical environment where Black people live, work, attend school, play, and pray—social deter-minants of health—have long had an outsized influence on health outcomes. And their impact became painfully obvious when the pandemic hit. Black Americans were more likely to be exposed to the virus. Segregation created crowded communities with multiple generations of family members, making social distancing and pro-tecting elders difficult. Black people were also more likely to be essential workers employed in service jobs—in transportation, government, health care, and food-supply services—as well as in low-wage or temporary jobs. Rather than telecommuting from home on Zoom, they were riding public transportation and working face-to-face, raising their risk of coming into contact with COVID. Unsurprisingly, the neighborhoods on the South Side of Chicago, where my mother was born and raised and where earlier in this book I mentioned that residents live thirty fewer years than their peers nine miles north, were the hardest hit as COVID raged.

Health-care facilities in Black communities are often crumbling or nonexistent, which, at the start of the pandemic especially, meant that people there were unable to find out if they had been infected with the virus, which made it difficult to protect themselves and others. Studies showed that white communities had more testing sites per capita than Black and Latinx ones, and some Black rural areas were labeled "testing deserts" because of the scarcity. As COVID rose to crisis proportions in Philadelphia, a local Black physician, Ala Stanford, MD, created DIY testing sites in Black communities. She recruited volunteer doctors, nurses, and med students and used her personal savings and donations collected through a GoFundMe campaign to test for COVID in church parking lots and in tents on street corners in Philly. Between April and October, her group, Black Doctors COVID-19 Consortium, tested more than ten thousand people.

The most recognizable social determinant of health is damage to the environment itself, and as scientists and policy makers have known since the 1980s, Black and poor communities live closest to polluting manufacturers and shoulder a disproportionate burden of the nation's dirty air. A paper released in April 2020 made an explicit link between air pollution and poor COVID-19 outcomes. Researchers at the Harvard T. H. Chan School of Public Health found that a majority of the conditions that increase the risk of death from COVID-19 are also worsened by long-term exposure to air pollution. After analyzing more than three thousand U.S. counties, the researchers concluded that even a small increase in exposure to fine particulate matter—tiny particles in the air—leads to a significant increase in the COVID-19 death rate.

The well-documented, long-standing bias and discrimination in health care also revealed itself during the pandemic. With a nod toward both the unequal impact of COVID-19 on African Americans and the history of discrimination in medical care, the CDC created a set of health equity principles to guide providers when treating patients of color during the pandemic. But racial bias baked into algorithms used to calibrate medical machines proved more difficult to avoid. Similar to the way racism has been embedded in the spirometer dating back to slavery, the pulse oximeter, a medical device used to measure oxygen levels in the blood of COVID-19 patients, has a design flaw that causes it to take inaccurate readings in African American patients. The device helps health-care providers gauge the severity of a coronavirus infection and decide whether to admit patients or send them home. A study published in December 2020 found that people with darker skin were three times more likely to receive misleading results. The test, which works using small beams of light that pass through the blood, was designed with white skin as the default.

But the case of Susan Moore, MD, provided the most observable and egregious example of the mash-up of COVID and racism in our current medical system. In late November 2020, Dr. Moore, a licensed physician in the Indianapolis area, would learn that years of medical training and credentials she worked hard to earn would fail to protect her from the medical system itself. On November 29, Dr. Moore tested positive for COVID-19 and checked herself into Indiana University Health North Hospital. On December 4, she posted a video on her Facebook page that showed her lying in her hospital bed, a breathing tube inserted in her nose. In the widely circulated video, she described disrespectful treatment by a white physician who rejected her plea for additional doses of a standard antiviral medication used to treat COVID. And despite what she described as excruciating pain, he told her he was "uncomfortable" giving her additional pain medication and tried to send her home. Through tears Dr. Moore said he made her feel like a drug addict. Looking directly into the camera, her voice laced with anger, Dr. Moore denounced the U.S. health-care system that had forsaken her: "I put forth and I maintain if I was white, I wouldn't have to go through that. This is how Black people get killed." Dr. Moore died two weeks later at age fifty-two. After her death, an external review concluded that Indiana University Health was not responsible for her death but that Dr. Moore's providers at the facility lacked "awareness of implicit racial bias" and stated that "there was a lack of empathy and compassion shown in the delivery of her care." An earlier statement from the president and CEO of the organization seemed to place blame for her death on Dr. Moore herself, explaining that the nursing staff at the facility might have been intimidated by her medical expertise.

When a COVID-19 vaccine was introduced to the public in 2021, predictably, Black people received fewer shares of vaccinations compared with other Americans. First, the vaccine was not consistently available in both rural and urban Black communities. Distribution relied on existing infrastructure, which was lacking in some predominantly Black areas. In Washington, D.C., 40 percent of early vaccine appointments were snapped up by residents of its wealthiest and primarily white ward, even though Black residents of the city accounted for 74 percent of deaths, 48 percent of cases, and nearly half of the population. A similar trend occurred in New York City, where I live. Disproportionate numbers of Black people were also wary of taking the vaccine, not trusting a medical system that had caused them harm dating back centuries. In December 2020, a poll released by the Kaiser Family Foundation showed that among racial and ethnic groups Black Americans were the most hesitant to get vaccinated against COVID. In the survey, more than one-third of African Americans said they would probably or definitely not get the vaccine even if it was determined to be safe by scientists and widely available for free. As with other medical studies, Black people were underrepresented in the clinical trials for the two initial COVID-19 vaccines produced by Pfizer and Moderna compared with their share of the population. The vast majority of the participants were white, even though Black people had worse outcomes from the disease.

The sickness and addiction I witnessed in West Virginia also intensified with COVID-19. Data compiled by the CDC showed a sharp rise in opioid deaths at the time when COVID lockdowns began in March 2020. Anxiety and despair over the pandemic might have contributed to greater drug use, and lockdowns made it challenging for people to receive in-person treatment for existing substance abuse problems. Social isolation made it more likely that people would use these substances alone, with less chance of a rescue in case of an accidental overdose. Increased drug use led to a spike in HIV transmission. In Kanawha County, West Virginia, where I visited in October 2020, the HIV outbreak expanded to crisis proportions during the pandemic. In early 2021, the chief of HIV prevention at the CDC called the outbreak of the virus in Kanawha "the most concerning in the United States." West Virginia's governor, Jim Justice, turned a blind eye to the surge of overdose deaths and HIV cases: in April 2021 he signed a bill that hampered harm-reduction efforts, making it harder to get clean needles.

Finally, the pandemic has exacted a toll on African Americans in ways that are less evident. Black people were more likely than other Americans to know someone who had contracted COVID and/or died of the virus. Nearly half of Black respondents in a survey conducted by the Commonwealth Fund reported experiencing an economic challenge because of the pandemic, substantially more than the 21 percent of white respondents. In the same poll, Black respondents reported pandemic-related mental health concerns at a rate approximately ten points higher than whites.

Still, I remain optimistic. After my May cover story on the New Orleans Zulu club and why COVID was hitting Black Americans so hard, I felt a profound shift in the level of receptiveness to its ideas. I was invited to present lectures and conduct workshops about inequality and health at least three dozen times—at Harvard, Yale, Howard, Northwestern, Tulane, UCLA, MIT, the CDC, and other agencies, community groups, and colleges. I also addressed journalism students and reporting fellows numerous times; they were hungry to understand how to cover racial health disparities, specifically how to interview "real people" like Nicole Charles with respect and empathy.

During these presentations I am often asked if I feel hopeful about the future. Without a second thought, I continue to answer yes. Together, America's racial reckoning and a pandemic that has exposed long-standing racial health inequality have thrown an accelerant on a slow-burning fire of awareness, forcing America to grapple with issues of race and justice and understand the origins of racism and its continued impact on the well-being of people and communities. My debate in February 2020 about whether my colleagues and I should explicitly label bias in the health-care system as racism in the title of our talk now seems like a lifetime ago. Just six months later it had become commonplace to call out racism as a public health threat, not only in the most progressive circles like Krieger's Spirit of 1848 forum, but in nearly every discussion of inequality and health. The theories of many racial health equity experts who have been toiling for decades, often behind the scenes, have been thrust into the limelight. David Williams and Arline Geronimus have seen their profiles rise and their theories and voices uplifted during the pandemic. Nancy Krieger was interviewed in *The New Yorker* in the spring, and despite those early rejections she had two dozen scientific studies and expert essays published about COVID in 2020, several with her colleague Mary Bassett. In response to the ill-treatment and ultimate death of Dr. Susan Moore, Joia Crear-Perry, Camara Jones, and Aletha Maybank teamed up with another Black female physician, Uché Blackstock, to write a scathing *Washington Post* editorial in December 2020 asking, "If a physician can't be heard by her own peers to save her life, then who will listen?" They titled their piece "Say Her Name," a callback to Breonna Taylor, the Black medical worker who was shot dead by a member of the Louisville Metro Police Department in March during a botched raid on her apartment. As with George Floyd, her death set off wide-scale demonstrations over policing and racial injustice.

Whereas in the past, race was considered a risk factor for a number of health conditions and early death, now it is clear that we must speak the harder truth: it's not race, something about being Black, or something wrong with the Black body, but racism that makes people sick and shortens their lives. Even after science finds a cure for COVID-19, racism in medicine is the harder virus to kill. But now is the time. The pandemic and the gross injustice of the state-involved killings of George Floyd, Breonna Taylor, and others have opened hearts and minds across the races to create an opportunity like no other to discuss and confront racism in America; now is the time to create transformative change in health, health care, and health equity in our nation. During the pandemic, California moved ahead of the country, requiring implicit bias training for health-care providers as part of their mandatory continuing education certification beginning in January 2022. The rest of the nation should follow suit.

I'd like to end with the words of Clyde W. Yancy, MD, chief of cardiology in the Department of Medicine at Northwestern's Feinberg School of Medicine. His essay on Black Americans and COVID-19 was published online in *The Journal of the American Medical Association* on April 15, which prompted me to interview him for my article about the Zulu club. As a boy growing up in Baton Rouge, Louisiana, and later as a student at Southern University and the Tulane University School of Medicine, Dr. Yancy remembers being fascinated with the decorated coconuts that were the sought-after prize of the Krewe of Zulu parade. During an interview he told me that that memory has been marred by his longtime study of racial health disparities and his knowledge of the unequal pain that has come to define the American outbreak of COVID-19. The tragedy of the Zulu members—and the larger heartbreak of the pandemic's effects on African Americans—must be a moment of epiphany, a wake-up call and call to action. We can no longer look away from the impact of the racial health disparities that have been part of the American story since the beginning of our nation. This is not how a just society treats a segment of its population. As Dr. Yancy said, "COVID-19 has taken off the Band-Aid that was covering the wound, pointed out how deep it is, and left us no other choice but to finally say, we get it, we see it."

ACKNOWLEDGMENTS

This book took me a long time to conceptualize, research, and write and is the culmination of years of thinking, reporting, and, especially, listening. It could not have come into the world without the faith and commitment of many people.

I am fortunate to have *The New York Times Magazine* as my home base, and I thank my colleagues for their own exceptional work and for getting my stories out of my head and onto the page. I am particularly grateful to be part of the 1619 Project, conceived by Nikole Hannah-Jones, which expanded my thinking. I extend special appreciation to my editor Jessica Lustig, who stays by my side every step of every story—with encouragement, attention to detail, long phone calls, and sparkling wine.

To the students, staff, and faculty at the Craig Newmark Graduate School of Journalism at CUNY and the City College of New York, thank you for showing me the importance of learning as you teach.

I am deeply indebted to a number of scientists, physicians, historians, and activists for their unshakable commitment to the ideas and concepts in the book. Thank you to Byllye Avery, Mary Bassett, Robert Bullard, Catherine Coleman Flowers, Harold Freeman, Vanessa Northington Gamble, Helene Gayle, Arline Geronimus, Evelynn Hammonds, Camara Jones, Nancy Krieger, Greg Millett, Dorothy Roberts, Loretta Ross, Harriet Washington, David Williams, and Phill Wilson for lighting my way.

I offer immense gratitude to everyone who shared their personal stories with me, peeling back the layers of your lives and sometimes your pain in order to lift up my work and make it relatable and meaningful. U-Meleni, your poetry leaves me breathless.

To my agent, Alia Hanna Habib—thank goodness you didn't listen when I insisted I didn't want to write a book. I am grateful to have you as my ride or die.

Many thanks to the team at Doubleday, especially Kris Puopolo, for your wisdom, careful reading, and hand-holding. Not only are you one of the finest editors in the business but also an attentive, patient collaborator. As an anxious writer, I extend gratitude to Julie Tate and Maryanne Warrick for your help with the details and to several others who supported me by fact-finding and organizing and in other invaluable ways—Shelby Boamah, Ayana Byrd, Avery Homer, Amari Leigh, Rachel Pride, and particularly Audrey Stewart, thank you.

My writer friends, who are very busy with their own work, took the time to offer encouragement, long walks, and longer talks: Allison Abner, Jeannine Amber, Hilary Beard, Andrea Bernstein, Sarah Broome, Benilde Little, Sarah Schulman, Liz Welch, and Teresa Wiltz, I appreciate you. Love to Laura Petrillo for weekly mental health check-ins.

To the Sunday dinner crew—Jackie, Juliet, Jane, Toshi R., Tashawn, Toshi G., and Jackson—I am grateful to you for food, family, and unfailing support. I could not ask for a better family. Mom, Alicia, Kali, Nic, Lorry, and Faye Michelle, I love you, I thank you. And, finally, to Jana—your unwavering belief in me and steady presence kept me going from the beginning of the process to the very end. Thank you for being there and for being you.

NOTES

CHAPTER ONE: EVERYTHING I THOUGHT WAS WRONG

1 Although the United States: Irene Papanicolas et al., "Health Care Spending in the United States and Other High-Income Countries," *Journal of the American Medical Association,* March 13, 2018, 1024–39, jamanetwork.com.

1 spends more on health care: Organisation for Economic Co-operation and Development, "Health Spending," accessed June 2021, data.oecd .org.

1 The United States has the highest rate: Organisation for Economic Co-operation and Development, "Infant Mortality Rates," accessed June 2021, data.oecd.org.

1 lowest life expectancy: Organisation for Economic Co-operation and Development, "Life Expectancy at Birth," accessed June 2021, data.oecd .org.

1 The health outcomes of Black Americans: Steven H. Woolf and Laudan Aron, eds., *U.S. Health in International Perspective: Shorter Lives, Poorer Health* (Washington, D.C.: National Academies Press, 2013).

1 At every stage of life: Centers for Disease Control and Prevention, "Impact of Racism on Our Nation's Health," April 8, 2021, www.cdc.gov.

1 Black babies are more than twice: Centers for Disease Control and Prevention, "Infant Mortality," Sept. 10, 2020, www.cdc.gov.

1 Black life expectancy: Centers for Disease Control and Prevention, "Health, United States, 2019—Data Finder," March 2, 2021, www.cdc .gov.

1 African Americans have elevated death rates: Timothy J. Cunningham et al., "Vital Signs: Racial Disparities in Age-Specific Mortality Among Blacks or African Americans—United States, 1999–2015," *Morbidity and Mortality Weekly Report,* May 5, 2017, www.cdc.gov.

2 In a phrase: Arline T. Geronimus et al., "Weathering, Drugs, and Whack-a-Mole: Fundamental and Proximate Causes of Widening Educational Inequity in U.S. Life Expectancy by Sex and Race, 1990–2015," *Journal of Health and Social Behavior* 60, no. 2 (2019): 222–39.

2 Even when income, education: Anne Case and Angus Deaton, "Life Expectancy in Adulthood Is Falling for Those Without a BA Degree, but as Educational Gaps Have Widened, Racial Gaps Have Narrowed," *Proceedings of the National Academy of Sciences of the United States of America,* March 16, 2021, www.pnas.org.

2 College-educated Black mothers: Samantha Artiga et al., "Racial Disparities in Maternal and Infant Health: An Overview," Kaiser Family Foundation, Nov. 10, 2020, www.kff.org.

3 The mission, instilled in everyone: *Essence,* "About," accessed June 2021, www.essence.com.

4 the Heckler Report: Margaret M. Heckler, *Report of the Secretary's Task Force on Black and Minority Health,* vol. 1, *Executive Summary* (Washington, D.C.: U.S. Department of Health and Human Services, 1985). In the Heckler Report, the Black-white health disparity was widest, but overall Blacks also fared worse than the other so-called minority groups—Hispanic, Asian/Pacific Islanders, and Native Americans. In fact, as an aggregate, Asian/Pacific Islanders were healthier and lived longer than all racial/ethnic groups, including whites. Still, the authors of the report noted "data deficiencies," including inadequate sample sizes for minorities other than Blacks, that made it difficult to create an accurate picture.

5 "Progress depends more on education": Marlene Cimons, "Need for Education, Behavior Changes Cited: Minorities Suffer from Health Gap," *Los Angeles Times,* Oct. 17, 1985, www.latimes.com.

5 "implication, of course, is that": Edith Irby Jones, "Closing the Health Status Gap for Blacks and Other Minorities," *Journal of the National Medical Association* 78, no. 6 (1986).

7 By the time I was: Ryan Marx, "Chicago Homicide Data Since 1957," *Chicago Tribune,* March 2, 2016, www.chicagotribune.com.

7 nearly a third of all Black residents: U.S. Department of Commerce, *Employment Profiles of Selected Low-Income Areas, Chicago, Ill.—Summary,* PHC (3)-16 (Washington, D.C.: U.S. Government Printing Office, 1972).

7 In the 1970s, the overall Black population: Neil J. Smelser et al., eds., *America Becoming: Racial Trends and Their Consequences* (Washington, D.C.: National Academy Press, 2001), 1:52.

10 co-written a groundbreaking article: Colin McCord and Harold P. Freeman, "Excess Mortality in Harlem," *New England Journal of Medicine,* Jan. 18, 1990, 173–77, www.nejm.org.

13 he had founded: Harold P. Freeman Patient Navigation Institute, hpfreemanpni.org.

13 In the Black community: Philip D. Curtin, "The Slavery Hypothesis for Hypertension Among African Americans: The Historical Evidence," *American Journal of Public Health* 82, no. 12 (Dec. 1992): 1681–86, ajph.aphapublications.org.

13 hypertension researcher Clarence Grim: Rozalynn S. Frazier, "'African Gene Theory' Is a Myth, and It's Harming Black Men's Heart Health," *Men's Health,* Jan. 24, 2021, www.menshealth.com.

13 This theory was so widespread: Osagie K. Obasogie, "Oprah's Unhealthy Mistake," *Los Angeles Times,* May 17, 2007, www.latimes.com.

13 "In people who have this gene": American Heart Association, "High Blood Pressure and African Americans," Oct. 31, 2016, www.heart.org.

16 the California Black Women's Health Project: Earlise C. Ward et al., "African American Women's Beliefs, Coping Behaviors, and Barriers to Seeking Mental Health Services," *Qualitative Health Research* 19, no. 11 (Nov. 2009): 1589–601.

16 "i found god in myself": Ntozake Shange, *For Colored Girls Who Have Considered Suicide When the Rainbow Is Enuf* (New York: Scribner, 2010), 87.

17 By then, research had mounted: Arline T. Geronimus, "The Weathering Hypothesis and the Health of African American Women and Infants: Evidence and Speculations," *Ethnicity and Disease* 2, no. 3 (Summer 1992): 207–21.

19 When the story, "The Hidden Toll": Linda Villarosa, "Why America's Black Mothers and Babies Are in a Life-or-Death Crisis," *New York Times Magazine,* April 11, 2018, www.nytimes.com. Print version titled "The Hidden Toll: Why America's Black Mothers and Babies Are in a Life-or-Death Crisis."

21 "We are the ones": Leandris C. Liburd, "'I'm Sick and Tired of Being Sick and Tired' (Fannie Lou Hamer, 1964)—Why We Work to Create Pathways to Health Equity," Centers for Disease Control, Conversations in Equity, April 30, 2015, blogs.cdc.gov.

21 "'our people, our problem'": Black AIDS Institute, accessed June 2021, blackaids.org.

CHAPTER TWO: THE DANGEROUS MYTH
THAT BLACK BODIES ARE DIFFERENT

22 The lawsuit *Relf v. Weinberger:* Southern Poverty Law Center, "Relf v. Weinberger," www.splcenter.org.

22 In his autobiography: J. Marion Sims, *The Story of My Life* (New York: D. Appleton, 1884), 236–37.

23 Almost a century later: Tuskegee University, "About the USPHS Syphilis Study," accessed June 2021, www.tuskegee.edu.

23 Recruitment flyers read: MaconHistory, "Tuskegee Syphilis Study," accessed June 2021, maconhistory.weebly.com. Author visited Tuskegee Center for Bioethics, where an original pamphlet was displayed.

23 "a notoriously syphilis-soaked race": James H. Jones, *Bad Blood: The Tuskegee Syphilis Experiment* (1981; New York: Free Press, 1993), 16.

23 Late in the era: Rebecca Skloot, *The Immortal Life of Henrietta Lacks* (New York: Crown, 2010).

23 In 1951, Lacks visited: Johns Hopkins Medicine, "The Legacy of Henrietta Lacks," accessed June 2021, www.hopkinsmedicine.org.

24 More than seventy years after: Amy Dockser Marcus, "Henrietta Lacks and Her Remarkable Cells Will Finally See Some Payback," *Wall Street Journal,* Aug. 1, 2020, www.wsj.com.

24 In 1973, Congress held hearings: Centers for Disease Control and Prevention, "The Tuskegee Timeline," accessed April 22, 2021, www.cdc.gov.

24 In 1997, when issuing a formal apology: White House Office of the Press Secretary, "Apology for Study Done in Tuskegee," May 16, 1997, clintonwhitehouse4.archives.gov.

24 In 2018, a statue celebrating: William Neuman, "City Orders Sims Statue Removed from Central Park," *New York Times,* April 16, 2018, www.nytimes.com; Esha Ray and Denis Slattery, "Protesters Demand Removal of Central Park Statue of 19th Century Doctor Who Experimented on Slave Women," *New York Daily News,* Aug. 20, 2017, www.nydailynews.com.

25 "I can show you": Relf sisters, interview by author, Montgomery, Ala., Dec. 17, 2018.

26 "I was waiting to see": Bly, interview by author, Montgomery, Ala., Feb. 29, 2020.

26 As she continued meeting: B. Drummond Ayres Jr., "Racism, Ethics, and Rights at Issue in Sterilization Case," *New York Times,* July 2, 1973, www.nytimes.com.

26 In 1910, 90 percent of all African Americans: "The Great Migration," History.com, Jan. 26, 2021, www.history.com.

26 Of those remaining in the South: Isabel Wilkerson, "The Long-Lasting Legacy of the Great Migration," *Smithsonian Magazine,* Sept. 2016, www.smithsonianmag.com; James N. Gregory, "The Second Great Migration: A Historical Overview," in *African American Urban History Since World War II,* ed. Kenneth L. Kusmer and Joe W. Trotter (Chicago: University of Chicago Press, 2009).

26 In Alabama specifically, census data: "Alabama's Population: 1800 to the Modern Era," AL.com, Dec. 28, 2019, www.al.com.

30 "I have amputated the legs": Benjamin Moseley, *A Treatise on Tropi-*

cal Diseases: And on the Climate of the West-Indies (London: G. G. and J. Robinson, 1795), 475.

30 "They have less hair": Thomas Jefferson, *Notes on the State of Virginia* (London, 1785).

31 In his widely read paper: Samuel Cartwright, "Report on the Diseases and Physical Peculiarities of the Negro Race," *New Orleans Medical and Surgical Journal,* May 1851.

33 Brown, who eventually managed to escape: John Brown, *Slave Life in Georgia: A Narrative of the Life, Sufferings, and Escape of John Brown, a Fugitive Slave, Now in England,* ed. L. A. Chamerovzow (London, 1855).

33 Cartwright was a professor: Lucius M. Lampton, "Samuel Adolphus Cartwright," *Mississippi Encyclopedia* (Jackson: Center for the Study of Southern Culture, University of Mississippi, 2017), mississippiencyclopedia .org.

33 specialized in illness and physiology: "Samuel Cartwright, Health and Physiology Committee of the Louisiana Medical Association," *Mississippi Encyclopedia,* 181.

34 The two attorneys had recently founded: Southern Poverty Law Center, "Our History," www.splcenter.org.

34 In July 1973, they filed: Law School Case Brief, *Relf v. Weinberger,* 372 F. Supp. 1196 (D.D.C. 1974), www.lexisnexis.com.

35 Just before the official filing: B. Drummond Ayres Jr., "Racism, Ethics, and Rights at Issue in Sterilization Case," *New York Times,* July 2, 1973, www.nytimes.com.

35 In a July 2, 1973, *New York Times* story: Ibid.

35 A *Times* article a few days later: B. Drummond Ayres Jr., "Sterilizing the Poor: Exploring Motives and Methods," *New York Times,* July 8, 1973, www.nytimes.com.

36 During the open hearing: Bill Kovach, "Sterilization Consent Not Given, Father Tells Kennedy's Panel," *New York Times,* July 11, 1973, www .nytimes.com.

37 At the Family Planning Clinic: Donna Franklin, "Beyond the Tuskegee Apology," *Washington Post,* May 29, 1997, www.washingtonpost.com.

37 Nial Ruth Cox: Edward Hudson, "Suit Seeks to Void Sterilization Law," *New York Times,* July 13, 1973, www.nytimes.com.

37 filed a suit: *Nial Ruth Cox, Appellant, v. A. M. Stanton, M.D., et al., Appellees,* No. 74-2218, U.S. Court of Appeals, Fourth Circuit, argued April 11, 1975 (decided Oct. 6, 1975), law.resource.org.

37 A governmental caseworker: Ria Tabacco Mar, "The Forgotten Time Ruth Bader Ginsburg Fought Against Forced Sterilization," *Washington Post,* Sept. 19, 2020, www.washingtonpost.com.

38 In North Carolina: "The Governor's Task Force to Determine the Method of Compensation for Victims of North Carolina's Eugenics Board," Jan. 27, 2012.

38 Like North Carolina, thirty-one other states: Lisa Ko, "Unwanted Sterilization and Eugenics Programs in the United States," *Independent Lens,* PBS, Jan. 29, 2016, www.pbs.org.

38 In California, more than 17,000: Nicole L. Novak et al., "Disproportionate Sterilization of Latinos Under California's Eugenic Sterilization Program, 1920–1945," *American Journal of Public Health* 108 (2018): 611–13, ajph.aphapublications.org.

38 In 1976, a study: National Library of Medicine, "1976: Government Admits Unauthorized Sterilization of Indian Women," www.nlm.nih.gov.

38 The same year, HEW reported: Eugenics Archive, "Puerto Rico," eugenicsarchive.ca.

38 Eventually, because of the Relfs' case: Southern Poverty Law Center, "Relf v. Weinberger."

39 they recruited Melvin Belli: Ayres, "Sterilizing the Poor, Exploring Motives and Methods."

39 Belli, nicknamed King of Torts: Richard Severo, "Melvin Belli Dies at 88; Flamboyant Lawyer Relished His Role as King of Torts," *New York Times,* July 11, 1996, www.nytimes.com.

39 To validate his theory: Lundy Braun, *Breathing Race into the Machine: The Surprising Career of the Spirometer from Plantation to Genetics* (Minneapolis: University of Minnesota Press, 2002). Dr. Braun's theory is summarized in Lundy Braun, "Race, Ethnicity, and Lung Function: A Brief History," *Canadian Journal of Respiratory Therapy* 51, no. 4 (Autumn 2015): 99–101.

40 A 2013 review of studies: Ronald Wyatt, "Pain and Ethnicity," *Virtual Mentor* 15, no. 5 (2013): 449–54.

40 As recently as 2016: Kelly M. Hoffman et al., "Racial Bias in Pain Assessment and Treatment Recommendations, and False Beliefs About Biological Differences Between Blacks and Whites," *Proceedings of the National Academy of Sciences of the United States of America* 113, no. 16 (2016): 4296–301, www.pnas.org.

41 Center for Investigative Reporting: Corey G. Johnson, "Female Inmates Sterilized in California Prisons Without Approval," *Reveal,* July 7, 2013, revealnews.org.

41 In 2017, Judge Sam Benningfield: "White County Inmates Given Reduced Jail Time if They Get Vasectomy," News Channel 5, Nashville, July 19, 2017, www.newschannel5.com.

41 In the fall of 2020: Caitlin Dickerson, Seth Freed Wessler, and Miriam Jordan, "Immigrants Say They Were Pressured into Unneeded Surgeries," *New York Times,* Sept. 29, 2020, www.nytimes.com.

42 "I felt sorry for them": Levin, phone interview by author, March 3, 2020.

42 In 2013, North Carolina: WFMY staff, "August 22, 1974: NC Woman's 'Forcibly Sterilized' Case Was Dismissed," WFMY News 2, Aug. 22, 2016, www.wfmynews2.com.

42 Virginia followed in 2015: Gary Robertson, "Virginia Lawmakers OK Payout to Forced Sterilization Survivors," Reuters, Feb. 26, 2015, www .reuters.com.

42 Though California apologized to the victims: Carl Ingram, "State Issues Apology for Policy of Sterilization," *Los Angeles Times,* March 12, 2003, www.latimes.com.

43 Their mother died in 1980: Minnie Relf obituary, *Montgomery Advertiser,* June 21, 1980, www.newspapers.com; Legacy.com, "Lonnie Relf," May 31, 2009, www.legacy.com.

CHAPTER THREE: UNEQUAL TREATMENT

44 *New York Times Magazine* cover story: Linda Villarosa, "Why America's Black Mothers and Babies Are in a Life-or-Death Crisis," *New York Times Magazine,* April 11, 2018, www.nytimes.com.

44 One Saturday afternoon: Center for Reproductive Rights, reproductiverights.org.

45 Her organization had recently collaborated: SisterSong, www.sistersong .net; Black Mamas Matter Alliance, blackmamasmatter.org.

45 "Did you know that a Black woman": Richard V. Reeves and Dayna Bowen Matthew, "6 Charts Showing the Race Gaps Within the American Middle Class," Brookings Institution, Oct. 21, 2016, www.brookings.edu.

46 At the Decolonizing Birth Conference: Decolonizing Birth Conference, www.decolonizingbirthconference.com.

46 By the end of the day: Birthmark Doulas, www.birthmarkdoulas.com.

46 This piece, part of Lost Mothers: Nina Martin and Renee Montagne, "The Last Person You Would Expect to Die in Childbirth," ProPublica and NPR, May 12, 2017, www.propublica.org; Nina Martin, Emma Cillekens, and Allessandra Freitas, "Lost Mothers," ProPublica, July 17, 2017, www.propublica.org.

47 In fact, as I was reporting: Corrine A. Riddell et al., "Trends in Differences in US Mortality Rates Between Black and White Infants," *JAMA Pediatrics* 71, no. 9 (Sept. 2017): 911–13, jamanetwork.com.

47 What's more, my friend: Dána-Ain Davis, *Reproductive Injustice: Racism, Pregnancy, and Premature Birth* (New York: New York University Press, 2019).

47 pointed me to statistics: Michael Haines, "Fertility and Mortality in the United States," Economic History Association, accessed June 17, 2021, eh .net.

48 Why is the current Black-white disparity: Reeves and Matthew, "6 Charts Showing the Race Gaps Within the American Middle Class."

48 studies out of Columbia University: Columbia University, Columbia Public Health, "Respectful Maternity Care," updated May 24, 2021, www.publichealth.columbia.edu.

49 Tanzania—where problems in pregnancy: World Health Organization, "Trends," accessed June 17, 2021, www.who.int/pmnch/activities/countries/tanzania/en/index1.html.

49 "There is something structural": Freedman, interview by author, Columbia University Mailman School of Public Health, Nov. 15, 2017.

49 "We don't do that here": Sang Hee Won (Lynn Freedman's colleague), phone interview by author, Feb. 28, 2017.

49 Landrum lived in Broadmoor: Greg B. Smith, "Neighborhood Effort Keeps Community Alive After Hurricane Katrina," *New York Daily News,* Aug. 22, 2015, www.nydailynews.com.

51 "Is she okay?": Landrum, interview by author, New Orleans, Nov. 2, 2017.

54 Rarely has an article: Kevin A. Schulman et al., "The Effect of Race and Sex on Physicians' Recommendation for Cardiac Catheterization," *New England Journal of Medicine,* Feb. 25, 1999, 618–26, www.nejm.org.

54 chose this topic for a reason: Centers for Disease Control and Prevention, "Facts About Hypertension," accessed Sept. 8, 2020, www.cdc.gov; Centers for Disease Control and Prevention, "Racial and Ethics Disparity in Heart Disease," *Health, United States Spotlight,* April 2019, www.cdc.gov.

54 majority of them white men: Avram Goldstein, "Race, Sex Disparity Found in Heart Care," *Washington Post,* Feb. 25, 1999, www.washingtonpost.com.

55 "How your doctor treats": Sally Satel, "The Indoctrinologists Are Coming," *Atlantic Monthly,* Jan. 2001.

55 "Last night we told you": Abigail Thernstrom and Stephan Thernstrom, eds., *Beyond the Color Line: New Perspectives on Race and Ethnicity in America* (Stanford, Calif.: Hoover Institution Press, 2001), 133.

55 "as close to a definition": Editorial, "Institutionalized Racism in Health Care," *Lancet* 9155 (1994): 765.

56 "serves to fuel anger": Lisa M. Schwartz, "Misunderstandings About the Effects of Race and Sex on Physicians' Referrals for Cardiac Catheterization," *New England Journal of Medicine,* July 22, 1999, 279–83, www.nejm.org.

56 Even as the controversy: Henry J. Kaiser Family Foundation, "Race, Ethnicity, and Medical Care: A Survey of Public Perceptions and Experiences," Oct. 1999, www.kff.org.

56 In 2000, Clinton signed legislation: National Institutes of Health, "National Institute on Minority Health and Health Disparities," *NIH Almanac,* accessed Dec. 4, 2020, www.nih.gov.

56 "When he was growing up": Schulman, Zoom interview by author, Aug. 4, 2020.

60 The Listening to Mothers: Listening to Mothers III Pregnancy and Birth, "Report of the Third National U.S. Survey of Women's Childbearing Experiences," May 2013, www.nationalpartnership.org.

61 National Academy of Sciences: National Academy of Sciences, "Mission," accessed June 18, 2021, www.nasonline.org.

61 *Unequal Treatment:* Brian D. Smedley, Adrienne Y. Stith, and Alan R. Nelson, eds., *Unequal Treatment: Confronting Racial and Ethnic Disparities in Health Care* (Washington, D.C.: National Academies Press, 2003). The report was released in March 2002 and published in 2003.

62 A mention of Dr. Kevin Schulman's: Thomas E. Perez, "The Civil Rights Dimension of Racial and Ethnic Disparities in Health Status," in Smedley, Stith, and Nelson, *Unequal Treatment.*

62 "To the extent that doctors": "Subtle Racism in Medicine," *New York Times,* March 22, 2002, www.nytimes.com.

63 Two weeks after the publication: Luis Ferré-Sadurní, "New York to Expand Use of Doulas to Reduce Childbirth Deaths," *New York Times,* April 22, 2018, www.nytimes.com.

63 Inspired by the story: Grace Douglas, "Award-Winning Journalist to Discuss the American Infant Mortality Crisis," *News @ ODU,* Old Dominion University, Jan. 21, 2020, www.odu.edu.

63 Merck announced: "Merck Announces 'Safer Childbirth Cities' Initiative, Issues Call to Action to Reverse the Rise in U.S. Maternal Deaths," Merck press release, Oct. 1, 2018, www.merck.com.

63 Most exciting for me: Louisiana Department of Health, Bureau of Family Health, "Louisiana Perinatal Quality Collaborative (LaPQC)," accessed June 18, 2021, ldh.la.gov.

65 In January 2018: Rob Haskell, "Serena Williams on Motherhood, Marriage, and Making Her Comeback," *Vogue,* Jan. 10, 2018, www.vogue.com.

CHAPTER FOUR: SOMETHING ABOUT BEING BLACK
IS BAD FOR YOUR BODY AND YOUR BABY

67 Their experiences support the findings: Richard David and James Collins Jr., "Disparities in Infant Mortality: What's Genetics Got to Do with It?," *American Journal of Public Health* 97, no. 7 (July 2007): 1191–97, ajph.aphapublications.org.

67 "Something about growing up": "Disparities in Infant Mortality Not Related to Race, Study Finds," *Science Daily,* July 31, 2007, www.sciencedaily.com.

70 Our country, the richest in the world: "Preterm Births Cost U.S. $26 Billion a Year; Multidisciplinary Research Effort Needed to Prevent Early Births," *National Academies of Sciences Engineering Medicine,* July 13, 2006, www.nationalacademies.org.

70 In general, in the United States: World Bank, "The Current Health Expenditure (% of GDP)," data.worldbank.org.

70 America spends nearly $11,000: World Bank, "Current Health Expenditure Per Capita (Current US$)," data.worldbank.org.

70 However, when the research pair: James Collins Jr. and Richard David, "The Differential Effect of Traditional Risk Factors on Infant Birthweight Among Blacks and Whites in Chicago," *American Journal of Public Health* 80, no. 6 (June 1990), ajph.aphapublications.org.

71 To test their theory: Richard J. David and James Collins Jr., "Differing Birth Weight Among Infants of U.S.-Born Blacks, African-Born Blacks, and U.S.-Born Whites," *New England Journal of Medicine,* Oct. 23, 1997, 1209–14, www.nejm.org.

71 For this study: James Collins Jr., Shou-Yien Wu, and Richard J. David, "Differing Intergenerational Birth Weights Among the Descendants of US-Born and Foreign-Born Whites and African Americans in Illinois," *American Journal of Epidemiology* 155, no. 3 (2002): 210–16.

71 Finally, in 2007, Drs. David and Collins: David and Collins, "Disparities in Infant Mortality."

73 It contained what is now considered: Kenneth C. Schoendorf et al., "Mortality Among Infants of Black as Compared with White College-Educated Parents," *New England Journal of Medicine,* June 4, 1992, 1522–26, www.nejm.org.

74 A team of female researchers: Boston University Sloane Epidemiology Center, "Black Women's Health Study," accessed June 21, 2021, www.bu.edu.

74 They were interested in looking: Nurses' Health Study, "The Nurses' Health Study and Nurses' Health Study II Are Among the Largest Investigations into the Risk Factors for Major Chronic Diseases in Women," accessed June 21, 2021, nurseshealthstudy.org.

76 The next day I googled him: David R. Williams, "Miles to Go Before We Sleep: Racial Inequities in Health," *Journal of Health and Social Behavior* 53, no. 3 (Sept. 2012): 279–95.

77 In 2011, writing: Ronald Howell, "Before Their Time," *Yale Alumni Magazine,* May/June 2011, yalealumnimagazine.com.

79 "If you were a woman": Miller, phone interviews by author, Nov. 18 and Dec. 11, 2020.

79 about 2.6 percent of physicians are Black women: Association of American Medical Colleges, "Diversity in Medicine, Facts and Figures 2019," www.aamc.org.

80 Geronimus, who coined the term: Arline T. Geronimus, "The Weathering Hypothesis and the Health of African American Women and Infants: Evidence and Speculations," *Ethnicity and Disease* 2, no. 3 (Summer 1992): 207–21.

81 Inspired by the book: Carol B. Stack, *All Our Kin: Strategies for Survival in a Black Community* (New York: Basic Books, 1997).

82 That year, in the journal: Arline T. Geronimus, "On Teenage Childbearing and Neonatal Mortality in the United States," *Population and Development Review* 13, no. 2 (June 1987): 245–79.

82 Karen Pittman, a Black sociologist: Tamar Lewin, "Studies Cause Confusion on Impact of Teen-Age Pregnancy," *New York Times,* March 7, 1990, www.nytimes.com.

83 Geronimus persisted: Geronimus, "Weathering Hypothesis and the Health of African American Women and Infants."

83 concept of John Henryism: S. A. James et al., "John Henryism and Blood Pressure Differences Among Black Men," *Journal of Behavioral Medicine* 6, no. 3 (Sept. 1983): 259–78.

84 For her 2006 study: Arline T. Geronimus et al., "'Weathering' and Age Patterns of Allostatic Load Scores Among Blacks and Whites in the United States," *American Journal of Public Health* 96, no. 5 (2006): 826–33, ajph.aphapublications.org.

84 "Breaking Point": U-Meleni Mhlaba-Adebo, *Soul Psalms* (Berkeley, Calif.: She Writes Press, 2016).

85 "By then, I was starting to understand": Mhlaba-Adebo, interview by author, Boston, Sept. 30, 2020.

86 "Have You Ever": U-Meleni Mhlaba-Adebo, "Have You Ever," Nov. 24, 2020, YouTube, www.youtube.com.

87 "Poem for Jabu": Mhlaba-Adebo, *Soul Psalms,* 65.

89 "Her body is a weapon": U-Meleni Mhlaba-Adebo, "Her Body Is a Weapon," u-meleni.com.

CHAPTER FIVE: WHERE YOU LIVE MATTERS

90 Danielle Bailey grew up: Danielle Bailey-Lash and Caroline Armijo, interviews by author, March 14, 2019.

90 a town of about fifteen hundred: U.S. Census Bureau, "Walnut Cove Town, North Carolina," www.census.gov.

91 Though a sign encourages fishing: A. Dennis Lemly, "Symptoms and Implications of Selenium Toxicity in Fish: The Belews Lake Case Example," *Aquatic Toxicology* 57 (2002): 39–49, www.fs.usda.gov.

91 In 2014, the danger became: Department of Environment and Natural Resources, "DENR Response to Duke Energy Coal Ash Spill," May 12, 2014, files.nc.gov.

91 Because the pond was unlined: Earthjustice, "Mapping the Coal Ash Contamination," Oct. 6, 2020, earthjustice.org.

92 Englewood High School, which: Illinois High School Glory Days, "Chicago Englewood High School 'Eagles,'" www.illinoishsglorydays.com.

92 about twenty-four thousand residents: Chicago Metropolitan Agency for Planning, "Englewood," June 2021, www.cmap.illinois.gov.

92 Today Chicago has the country's: "Large Life Expectancy Gaps in U.S. Cities Linked to Racial & Ethnic Segregation by Neighborhood," *NYU Langone Health News Hub,* June 5, 2019, nyulangone.org.

93 A wide-ranging report: NAACP, "Fumes Across the Fence-Line: The

Health Impacts of Air Pollution from Oil & Gas Facilities on African American Communities," Nov. 2017, naacp.org.

93 A study conducted by the EPA's: Ihab Mikati et al., "Disparities in Distribution of Particulate Matter Emission Sources by Race and Poverty Status," *American Journal of Public Health,* March 7, 2018, 480–85, ajph .aphapublications.org.

93 Ironically, another study: Christopher W. Tessum et al., "Inequity in Consumption of Goods and Services Adds to Racial–Ethnic Disparities in Air Pollution Exposure," *Proceedings of the National Academy of Sciences of the United States of America* 116, no. 13 (March 2019): 6001–6, www.pnas.org.

94 In December 2017: Mark D. Risser and Michael F. Wehner, "Attributable Human-Induced Changes in the Likelihood and Magnitude of the Observed Extreme Precipitation During Hurricane Harvey," *Geophysical Research Letters* 44, no. 24 (Dec. 2017): 12457–64, agupubs.onlinelibrary .wiley.com.

94 A 2017 survey: Megan L. McKenna et al., "Human Intestinal Parasite Burden and Poor Sanitation in Rural Alabama," *American Journal of Tropical Medicine and Hygiene* 97, no. 5 (2017): 1623–28, www.ajtmh .org; article corrected in *American Journal of Tropical Medicine and Hygiene* 98, no. 3 (March 2018): 936.

94 In 2017, a United Nations official: Connor Sheets, "UN Poverty Official Touring Alabama's Black Belt: 'I Haven't Seen This' in the First World," AL.com, Dec. 8, 2017, updated March 7, 2019, www.al.com.

Catherine Coleman Flowers, a MacArthur genius, wrote a book called *Waste: One Woman's Fight Against America's Dirty Secret* about Lowndes County, where she was born and raised.

95 "Call Tony and have him": Sandra Thomas, interview by author, Walnut Grove, N.C., Feb. 22, 2020.

96 Though cancer is an unpredictable: American Association of Neurological Surgeons, "Glioblastoma Multiforme," accessed June 28, 2021, www .aans.org.

96 Eventually, she discovered: Earthjustice, "Coal Ash Contaminates Our Lives," accessed June 28, 2021, earthjustice.org.

96 Seventy percent of coal ash ponds: Statement, Lisa Evans to U.S. Commission on Civil Rights, "Coal Ash Pollution and Impacts on Minority and Low-Income Communities," Jan. 22, 2016, www.dropbox.com/ s/g1ubwsnu4lye4v9/Evans%20USCCR%20statement%20010816.pdf ?dl=0.

96 North Carolina had more than one hundred: Lisa Sorg, "Do You Live near a Coal Ash Disposal Site?," *NC Policy Watch,* Sept. 4, 2018, www .ncpolicywatch.com.

97 Two years later, the state would admit: Michael Biesecker, "NC Toxicolo-

gists: Water near Duke's Dump Not Safe to Drink," Associated Press, Aug. 2, 2016, apnews.com.

98 This event, which received: Catherine E. Shoichet, "Spill Spews Tons of Coal Ash into North Carolina River," CNN, Feb. 9, 2014, www.cnn .com.

98 In 1896, when African Americans: Frederick L. Hoffman, *Race Traits and Tendencies of the American Negro* (New York: Macmillan, 1896).

99 Du Bois and his team: W. E. B. Du Bois and Isabel Eaton, *The Philadelphia Negro: A Social Study* (Philadelphia: Ginn, 1899; Philadelphia: University of Pennsylvania Press, 1996).

99 In a later work: W. E. Burghardt Du Bois, "The Health and Physique of the Negro American," *American Journal of Public Health* 93, no. 2 (Feb. 2003): 272–76. Journal article is excerpted from Du Bois, *The Health and Physique of the Negro American* (Atlanta: Atlanta University Press, 1906).

100 Even educated, affluent Blacks: Lewis Mumford Center for Comparative Urban and Regional Research University at Albany, "Separate and Unequal: The Neighborhood Gap for Blacks and Hispanics in Metropolitan America," Oct. 13, 2002, mumford.albany.edu.

100 Only 44 percent of Black Americans: Dana Anderson, "Minneapolis, Milwaukee & Salt Lake City Have the Lowest Black Homeownership Rates in the U.S., with Just One-Quarter of Black Families Owning Their Home," *Redfin News,* June 29, 2020, updated Oct. 19, 2020, www .redfin.com.

100 compared with about 65 percent: Census.gov, "Quarterly Residential Vacancies and Homeownership, First Quarter 2021," Release Number CB21-56, April 27, 2021, www.census.gov.

100 Homeownership, a pillar of the so-called American dream: Troy McMullen, "The 'Heartbreaking' Decrease in Black Homeownership," *Washington Post,* Feb. 28, 2019, www.washingtonpost.com.

100 This contributes to a wealth gap: Neil Bhutta et al., "Disparities in Wealth by Race and Ethnicity in the 2019 Survey of Consumer Finances," *Feds Notes,* Sept. 28, 2020, www.federalreserve.gov.

100 Many areas where the streets: Richard Rothstein, *The Color of Law* (New York: Liveright, 2018).

101 A 2020 study: National Community Reinvestment Coalition, "Redlining and Neighborhood Health," accessed June 29, 2021, ncrc.org.

101 According to the 2019 report: Samuel DuBois Cook Center on Social Equity, "The Plunder of Black Wealth in Chicago: New Findings on the Lasting Toll of Predatory Housing Contracts," May 2019, socialequity .duke.edu.

102 In 1978, Robert Bullard: Author interviews, phone June 21, 2018, and at the Climate Reality Leadership Corps Training, Atlanta, March 16, 2019.

102 The suit charged: Robert D. Bullard, "The Mountains of Houston: Environmental Justice and the Politics of Garbage" (2014), ricedesignalliance .org.

104 In his 1990 book: Robert D. Bullard, *Dumping in Dixie: Race, Class, and Environmental Quality* (Boulder, Colo.: Westview Press, 1990).

104 As Bullard was writing: Matt Reimann, "The EPA Chose This County for a Toxic Dump Because Its Residents Were 'Few, Black, and Poor,'" *Timeline,* April 3, 2017, timeline.com.

104 The study, *Toxic Wastes:* Commission for Racial Justice, United Church of Christ, *Toxic Wastes and Race in the United States* (1987), nrc.gov.

105 In 2007, the UCC revisited: Robert Bullard et al., *Toxic Wastes and Race at Twenty, 1987–2007,* United Church of Christ Justice and Witness Ministries, March 2007, www.nrdc.org.

105 In time for Black History Month: United Church of Christ, *"Breath to the People": Sacred Air and Toxic Pollution,* Feb. 2020, www.ucc.org.

106 In 1992, the EPA created: U.S. Environmental Protection Agency, "Environmental Justice Fact Sheet," April 1996, www.epa.gov.

106 The new office hired: Ali, interview by author at the Climate Reality Leadership Corps Training, Atlanta, March 16, 2019.

106 In 1994, the newly elected president: U.S. Environmental Protection Agency, "Laws and Regulations, Summary of Executive Order 12898—Federal Actions to Address Environmental Justice in Minority Populations and Low-Income Populations," Feb. 16, 1994, www.epa.gov.

107 Then, in 2017, Donald Trump: Juliet Eilperin and Brady Dennis, "White House Eyes Plan to Cut EPA Staff by One-Fifth, Eliminating Key Programs," *Washington Post,* March 1, 2017, www.washingtonpost.com.

107 The proposal also called for: Brady Dennis, "EPA Environmental Justice Leader Resigns, amid White House Plans to Dismantle Program," *Washington Post,* March 9, 2017, www.washingtonpost.com.

107 His three-page, single-spaced: Mustafa Santiago Ali resignation letter, March 8, 2017, www.documentcloud.org/documents/3514958-Final -Resignation-Letter-for-Administrator.html.

108 A year and a half later: Coral Davenport, Lisa Friedman, and Maggie Haberman, "E.P.A. Chief Scott Pruitt Resigns Under a Cloud of Ethics Scandals," *New York Times,* July 5, 2018, www.nytimes.com.

108 Before Pruitt was pushed out: Ihab Mikati et al., "Disparities in Distribution of Particulate Matter Emission Sources by Race and Poverty Status," *American Journal of Public Health,* March 7, 2018, 480–85, ajph .aphapublications.org.

108 The campaign outline states: Poor People's Campaign, "Our Demands," accessed June 29, 2021, www.poorpeoplescampaign.org.

109 The week after the North Carolina: Lisa Friedman, "Cost of New E.P.A. Coal Rules: Up to 1,400 New Deaths a Year," *New York Times,* Aug. 21, 2018, www.nytimes.com.

109 On that day, which was: "Danielle Bailey-Lash Comments 2018 Event," YouTube, www.youtube.com.

109 "If the coal ash": Amanda Dodson, "Al Gore Stops in Stokes County," *Stokes News,* Aug. 15, 2018, www.thestokesnews.com.

110 On Thursday, March 14: Climate Reality Project, "Three Great Moments from Our Atlanta Training," April 6, 2019, www.climaterealityproject .org.

111 on April 1, the North Carolina: North Carolina Environmental Quality, "DEQ Orders Duke Energy to Excavate Coal Ash at Six Remaining Sites," press release, April 1, 2019, deq.nc.gov.

111 The good news was short-lived: Lisa Sorg, "Duke Energy to DEQ: See you in court," *The Pulse,* NC Policy Watch, April 12, 2019, www.pulse .ncpolicywatch.org.

111 That means that though some notable Black: Charlotte Alter, Suyin Haynes, and Justin Worland, "Time 2019 Person of the Year, Greta Thunberg," *Time,* Dec. 23/Dec. 30, 2019, time.com.

112 In March 1990, more than a hundred: Southwest Organizing Project, Letter, March 16, 1990, www.ejnet.org.

112 The weekend event in 1991: Environmental Justice/Environmental Racism 17-point platform adopted at the First National People of Color Environmental Leadership Summit, Oct. 24–27, 1991, www.ejnet.org.

112 Bullard, one of the organizers: Deep South Center for Environmental Justice, "HBCU Climate Change Consortium," accessed June 30, 2021, www.dscej.org.

113 A 2018 survey: Dorceta E. Taylor, "Diversity in Environmental Organizations Reporting and Transparency Report No. 1," Jan. 2018, www .researchgate.net.

113 A 2019 report: Green 2.0, "Leaking Talent," accessed June 30, 2021, diversegreen.org.

114 The company reached a settlement: *Duke Energy Carolinas, LLC, and Duke Energy Progress, LLC, v. North Carolina Department of Environmental Quality,* settlement agreement, Dec. 31, 2019, www.southernenvironment.org.

114 Caroline thinks about her friend: Caroline Armijo, interviews by author, Stokes County, N.C., Feb. 21–23, 2020.

114 In 2018, inspired by Danielle: Lilies Project, Addressing Coal Ash Through Arts & Parks, accessed June 30, 2021, theliliesproject.org.

CHAPTER SIX: STRONG, LOUD, AND ANGRY: THE
INVISIBILITY OF BLACK EMOTIONAL PAIN

116 On a hectic day: Audrey Brianne, Zoom interview by author, March 20, 2021.

117 A 2018 national survey: Substance Abuse and Mental Health Services Administration, U.S. Department of Health and Human Services, "2018

National Survey on Drug Use and Health: African Americans," www
.samhsa.gov.

117 The proliferation of high-profile: Jacob Bor et al., "Police Killings and
Their Spillover Effects on the Mental Health of Black Americans: A Population Based, Quasi-experimental Study," *Lancet* 392 (2018): 302–10,
www.thelancet.com.

118 Instead, they are much more likely: V. A. Hiday et al., "Criminal Vic-
timization of Persons with Severe Mental Illness," *Psychiatric Services* 50
(Jan. 1999): 62–68.

118 A 2012 report: E. Fuller Torrey et al., "No Room at the Inn: Trends and
Consequences of Closing Public Psychiatric Hospitals, 2005–2010,"
Treatment Advocacy Center, July 19, 2012, www.treatmentadvocacycenter
.org.

118 In Zora Neale Hurston's: Zora Neale Hurston, *Their Eyes Were Watching
God* (New York: HarperCollins, 2021).

119 A 2009 study found: "Black Girls Are 50 Percent More Likely to Be
Bulimic Than White Girls," *Science Daily,* March 25, 2009, www
.sciencedaily.com.

119 A 2020 review of thirty-eight previous: Rachel W. Goode et al., "Binge
Eating and Binge-Eating Disorder in Black Women: A Systematic
Review," *International Journal of Eating Disorders* 53, no. 4 (April 2020):
491–507, onlinelibrary.wiley.com.

120 despite research that points to: Yunyu Xiao et al., "Temporal Trends
in Suicidal Ideation and Attempts Among US Adolescents by Sex and
Race/Ethnicity, 1991–2019," *JAMA Newtork Open* 4, no. 6 (June 2021),
www.jamanetwork.com.

120 McClain had first gained: Leanita McClain, "The Middle-Class Black's
Burden," *Newsweek,* Oct. 13, 1980, 12.

121 Her early poetry: Leanita McClain, *A Foot in Each World: Essays and Articles* (Evanston, Ill.: Northwestern University Press, 1986).

122 a very popular book: Terrie M. Williams, *Black Pain: It Just Looks Like
We're Not Hurting: Real Talk for When There's Nowhere to Go but Up* (New
York: Scribner, 2009).

123 Millions of African Americans: Mental Health America, "Black and African American Communities and Mental Health," accessed July 2, 2021,
www.mhanational.org; National Institute of Mental Health, "Mental
Health Information, Statistics," accessed July 2, 2021, www.nimh.nih
.gov.

123 about 84 percent of the psychology: "Psychology's Workforce Is Becoming More Diverse," *Monitor on Psychology* 51, no. 8 (2020): 19, www.apa
.org.

123 This includes Black people: Black Women's Health Imperative, "Postpartum Depression While Black," April 20, 2018, bwhi.org.

123 Mistreatment of African Americans: Alexander Thomas and Samuel Sillen, *Racism and Psychiatry* (New York: Carol, 1993).

123 A 1968 article: Walter Bromberg and Franck Simon, "The 'Protest' Psychosis: A Special Type of Reactive Psychosis," *Archives of General Psychiatry* 19, no. 2 (1968): 155–60, jamanetwork.com.

124 Black men are still four times: "African Americans More Likely to Be Misdiagnosed with Schizophrenia, Study Finds," *Science Daily,* March 21, 2019, www.sciencedaily.com.

124 Instead, according to a 2019 study: Michael A. Lindsey et al., "Trends of Suicidal Behaviors Among High School Students in the United States, 1991–2017," *Pediatrics* 144, no. 5 (Nov. 2019), pediatrics.aappublications .org.

125 Over Labor Day weekend: Gloria McMullen, interviews with author, Middletown, Conn., Aug. 10 and 22, 2020.

127 Forty percent of adults: Carolyn Zezima, "Incarcerated with Mental Illness: How to Reduce the Number of People with Mental Health Issues in Prison," *Psycom,* Aug. 12, 2020, www.psycom.net.

127 Individuals with severe mental illnesses: Doris A. Fuller et al., "Overlooked in the Undercounted: The Role of Mental Illness in Fatal Law Enforcement Encounters," Treatment Advocacy Center, Office of Research and Public Affairs, Dec. 2015, www.treatmentadvocacycenter.org.

127 Jails and prisons hold more people: E. Fuller Torrey et al., "More Mentally Ill Persons Are in Jails and Prisons Than Hospitals: A Survey of the States," Treatment Advocacy Center, May 2010, www.treatmentadvocacycenter .org.

127 By all accounts, including databases: Washington Post staff, "Fatal Force," *Washington Post,* updated July 2, 2021, www.washingtonpost .com; Guardian staff, "The Counted, People Killed by Police in the US," *Guardian,* accessed July 2, 2021, www.theguardian.com.

127 one in four fatal encounters: Fuller et al., "Overlooked in the Undercounted."

127 According to Mapping Police Violence: Mapping Police Violence, accessed July 3, 2021, mappingpoliceviolence.org.

128 "We would hear him": Karen McMullen, interview by author, Brooklyn, July 27, 2020.

132 Bipolar disorder, a brain condition: "Bipolar Disorder (Manic Depressive Illness)," Mental Illness Policy Organization, accessed July 3, 2021, mentalillnesspolicy.org.

132 Black people were not diagnosed properly: Kaja R. Johnson and Sheri L. Johnson, "Inadequate Treatment of Black Americans with Bipolar Disorder," *Psychiatric Services* 65, no. 2 (Feb. 2014): 255–58, ps.psychiatryonline .org.

134 While Black adults in the United States: Human Rights Watch, "US:

Disastrous Toll of Criminalizing Drug Use," Oct. 12, 2016, www.hrw .org; Tess Borden et al., *Every 25 Seconds: The Human Toll of Criminalizing Drug Use in the United States,* Human Rights Watch and American Civil Liberties Union, Oct. 2016, www.hrw.org.

134 In 1971, President Nixon: Equal Justice Initiative, "Nixon Adviser Admits War on Drugs Was Designed to Criminalize Black People," March 25, 2016, eji.org.

134 The kicker: Josh Rovner, "Racial Disparities in Youth Incarceration Persist," Sentencing Project, Feb. 3, 2021, www.sentencingproject.org.

134 In 1986, the Anti–Drug Abuse Act: American Civil Liberties Union, "Cracks in the System: 20 Years of the Unjust Federal Crack Cocaine Law," Oct. 2006, www.aclu.org.

134 Decades after the fact: Dan Baum, "Legalize It All," *Harper's Magazine,* April 2016, harpers.org.

135 2010 Fair Sentencing Act: American Civil Liberties Union, "Fair Sentencing Act," accessed July 3, 2021, www.aclu.org.

135 In fact, a 2017 analysis: Julie Netherland and Helena B. Hansen, "The War on Drugs That Wasn't: Wasted Whiteness, 'Dirty Doctors,' and Race in Media Coverage of Prescription Opioid Use," *Culture Medicine and Psychology* 40, no. 4 (Dec. 2016): 664–86; Yardena Schwartz, "Painkiller Use Breeds New Face of Heroin Addiction," NBC News, June 19, 2012, www.nbcnews.com.

135 Federal spending also reveals: Shannon Mullen et al., "Crack vs. Heroin," *Asbury Park Press,* Dec. 2, 2019, updated June 17, 2020, www.app.com.

137 According to the police report: McMullen Boston PD initial report, requested on Dec. 2, 2011; Commonwealth of Massachusetts Plymouth County Office of the District Attorney, "Investigation Concluded," Feb. 28, 2011.

139 Pressured into conducting an inquest: Commonwealth of Massachusetts Plymouth County Office of the District Attorney, "Investigation Concluded," Feb. 28, 2011.

139 Six years after his death: "The Schroeder Brothers Memorial Medal, the Department Medal of Honor, the Boston Police Relief Association Memorial Award," *Blackstonian,* Jan. 4, 2013, blackstonian.org.

CHAPTER SEVEN: DISCRIMINATION AND
ILL-TREATMENT CAN HARM EVERY BODY

141 Charlene Marshall: Erin Beck, "Banned from Attending White Colleges in 1950s, Former Delegate to Receive Honorary Degree," *Charleston Gazette-Mail,* May 15, 2015, www.wvgazettemail.com.

142 Ashley and Jason turn: Ashley and Jason (last names withheld), interview by author, Morgantown, W.Va., Oct. 26, 2020.

143 The other options that the Bartlett House: Bartlett Housing Solutions, "Our Programs," accessed July 26, 2021, www.bartletthousingsolutions.org.

143 Many of the Bartlett House clients: Department of Numbers, "Morgantown, West Virginia Unemployment," www.deptofnumbers.com.

144 But the census points to: U.S. Census Bureau, "Quick Facts Morgantown City, West Virginia," July 1, 2019, www.census.gov.

144 That means that most: West Virginia Division of Labor, "Minimum Wage & Maximum Hours," accessed July 26, 2021, labor.wv.gov.

144 The local government's annual: "FY 2020 Annual Action Plan— Substantial Amendment, City of Morgantown, WV," Nov. 18, 2020, 61, www.morgantownwv.gov.

144 About a block up: West Virginia University, "WVU Facts," accessed July 26, 2021, www.wvu.edu.

146 That question sent me: U.S. Census Bureau. "Quick Facts West Virginia," July 1, 2019, www.census.gov.

146 West Virginia is part of Appalachia: Appalachian Regional Commission, "About the Appalachian Region," accessed July 26, 2021, www.arc.gov.

146 It has among the country's highest: Kaiser Family Foundation, "Poverty Rate by Race/Ethnicity" (2019), www.kff.org; John Deskins, "Human Capital in West Virginia," *West Virginia Executive,* March 4, 2020, www.wvexecutive.com.

146 Mining jobs peaked: Ken Ward Jr., "The Coal Industry Extracted a Steep Price from West Virginia. Now Natural Gas Is Leading the State Down the Same Path," ProPublica, April 27, 2018, www.propublica.org.

146 Ironically, one of the poorest states: Giacomo Tognini, "Not Just Trump and Bloomberg: Here Are the Billionaire Politicians of the Decade," *Forbes,* Dec. 26, 2019, www.forbes.com.

147 Along with Donald Trump: Tim Loh, "Governor Says Trump Interested in His Plan to Prop Up Coal Mining," Bloomberg, Aug. 9, 2017, www.bloomberg.com.

147 The state had the lowest life expectancy: Elizabeth Arias et al., "U.S. State Life Tables, 2018," *National Vital Statistics Reports* 70, no. 1 (March 2021), www.cdc.gov.

147 Racial health disparities: Louise Norris, "West Virginia and the ACA's Medicaid Expansion," healthinsurance.org, Oct. 16, 2020, www.healthinsurance.org; Jennifer Welsh, "Race and Life Expectancy in All 50 States," *Live Science,* March 5, 2012, www.livescience.com.

147 Still, it is worth examining: Steven H. Woolf and Heidi Schoomaker, "Life Expectancy and Mortality Rates in the United States, 1959–2017," *Journal of the American Medical Association,* Nov. 26, 2019, 1996–2016.

147 This, even though West Virginia expanded: Norris, "West Virginia and the ACA's Medicaid Expansion."

147 The obesity rate: West Virginia Department of Health and Human Resources, Bureau for Public Health, "Fast Facts" (2018), dhhr.wv.gov.

147 These health problems: Anne Case and Angus Deaton, "Mortality and Morbidity in the 21st Century," *Brookings Papers on Economic Activity* (Spring 2017), www.brookings.edu.

148 His 2016 best seller: J. D. Vance, *Hillbilly Elegy* (New York: HarperCollins, 2016).

148 what W. E. B. Du Bois described: W. E. B. Du Bois and Isabel Eaton, *The Philadelphia Negro: A Social Study* (Philadelphia: Ginn, 1899; Philadelphia: University of Pennsylvania Press, 1996).

148 "I need a haircut": Scott (last name withheld), interview by author, Morgantown, W.Va., Oct. 27, 2020.

149 Several years ago, Nicole Novak: Novak, interview by author, Iowa City, Iowa, Dec. 18, 2019.

150 The study, published in 2017: Nicole Novak et al., "Change in Birth Outcomes Among Infants Born to Latina Mothers After a Major Immigration Raid," *International Journal of Epidemiology* 46, no. 3 (June 2017): 839–49.

151 Caitlin Sussman, the Friendship House's: Caitlin Sussman, interview by author, Morgantown, W.Va., Oct. 26, 2020.

151 Nearly every U.S. media outlet: Anne Case and Angus Deaton, "Rising Morbidity and Mortality in Midlife Among White Non-Hispanic Americans in the 21st Century," *Proceedings of the National Academy of Sciences of the United States of America* 112, no. 49 (2015): 15078–83, pnas.org.

152 Between 1997, just after Purdue Pharma: Neil Davey, "Congress Must Do More to Address the U.S. Opioid Epidemic," Center for American Progress, Aug. 25, 2016, www.americanprogress.org.

152 But in 2007, the government cracked down: Barry Meier, "In Guilty Plea, OxyContin Maker to Pay $600 Million," *New York Times,* May 10, 2007, www.nytimes.com.

152 The vast majority of heroin users: "Prescription Opioids and Heroin Research Report, Prescription Opioid Use Is a Risk Factor for Heroin Use," National Institute on Drug Abuse, Oct. 1, 2015, www.drugabuse.gov.

152 Though Purdue Pharma pleaded: Meier, "In Guilty Plea, OxyContin Maker to Pay $600 Million."

153 Geronimus, while acknowledging: Arline Geronimus, interview by author, New York, Dec. 7, 2019.

153 Many are the Americans: Anne Case and Angus Deaton, *Deaths of Despair and the Future of Capitalism* (Princeton, N.J.: Princeton University Press, 2020), 38.

154 "This is where I'm going to put you": Dani Ludwig, interview by author, Morgantown, W.Va., Oct. 26, 2020.

155 He moved into Diamond Village: Daniel (last name withheld), interview by author, Morgantown, W.Va., Oct. 26, 2020.

156 "I know you're wondering": Paula (last name withheld), interview by author, Morgantown, W.Va., Oct. 26, 2020.

156 A thick paperback: Elizabeth Lesser, *Broken Open: How Difficult Times Can Help Us Grow* (New York: Ballantine Books, 2020).

156 On October 27, 2020: Morgantown Police Department, "Morgantown Police Respond to Drug Overdose," Oct. 2020, morgantownwv.gov.

157 A month later: Joe Buchanan, "City of Morgantown Clears Diamond Village Homeless Encampment," WDTV, Dec. 1, 2020, www.wdtv .com.

157 Between 2007 and 2012: Eric Eyre, "Drug Firms Poured 780M Painkillers into WV amid Rise of Overdoses," *Charleston Gazette-Mail,* Dec. 17, 2016, updated Dec. 27, 2017, www.wvgazettemail.com.

157 This led to an outbreak: Gregg S. Gonsalves and Forrest W. Crawford, "Dynamics of the HIV Outbreak and Response in Scott County, Indiana, 2011–2015: A Modeling Study," *Lancet HIV* 5, no. 10 (Oct. 2018): e569—e577.

157 In 2015, worried officials: Sean T. Allen et al., "Understanding the Public Health Consequences of Suspending a Rural Syringe Services Program: A Qualitative Study of the Experiences of People Who Inject Drugs," *Harm Reduction Journal* 16, no. 33 (2019), harmreductionjournal.biomedcentral .com.

157 Several decades of research: Centers for Disease Control and Prevention, "Summary of Information on the Safety and Effectiveness of Syringe Services Programs (SSPs)," accessed May 23, 2019, www.cdc.gov.

158 At its peak, nearly five hundred: Josh Katz, "Why a City at the Center of the Opioid Crisis Gave Up a Tool to Fight It," *New York Times,* April 27, 2018, www.nytimes.com.

158 "mini-mall for junkies and drug dealers": Ibid.

158 The group was considering: Leslie Rubin, "EXCLUSIVE: Charleston Police Launch Investigation into Off-the-Radar Needle Distribution," WCHS, Oct. 22, 2020, wchstv.com.

CHAPTER EIGHT: PUTTING THE CARE
BACK IN HEALTH CARE: SOLUTIONS

163 By the time the story ran: Linda Villarosa and Joan Roberts, "Nobody's Safe," *Essence,* June 1987.

163 In November 1996: Andrew Sullivan, "When Plagues End," *New York Times Magazine,* Nov. 10, 1996, www.nytimes.com.

163 A month later: Newsweek staff, "The End of Aids?," *Newsweek,* Dec. 1, 1996, www.newsweek.com.

163 HIV had been framed: Centers for Disease Control and Prevention, "U.S. HIV and AIDS Cases Reported Through December 1996," *HIV/AIDS Surveillance Report* 8, no. 2 (Dec. 1996), www.cdc.gov.

164 The first, "AIDS Fears Grow": Linda Villarosa, "AIDS Fears Grow for Black Women," *New York Times,* April 5, 2004, www.nytimes.com.

164 The second, "Patients with H.I.V.": Linda Villarosa, "Patients with H.I.V. Seen as Separated by a Racial Divide," *New York Times,* Aug. 7, 2004, www.nytimes.com.

164 In 2016, now nearly thirty years: Centers for Disease Control and Prevention, "Lifetime Risk of HIV Diagnosis, Half of Black Gay Men and a Quarter of Latino Men Projected to Be Diagnosed Within Their Lifetime," *NCHHSTP Newsroom,* Feb. 23, 2016, www.cdc.gov.

164 Ground zero was Jackson: Eli Samuel Rosenberg et al., "Rates of Prevalent HIV Infection, Prevalent Diagnoses, and New Diagnoses Among Men Who Have Sex with Men in US States, Metropolitan Statistical Areas, and Counties, 2012–2013," *Journal of Medical Internet Research* 2, no. 1 (2016), publichealth.jmir.org.

165 The story, which ran on the cover: Linda Villarosa, "America's Hidden H.I.V. Epidemic," *New York Times Magazine,* June 6, 2017, www.nytimes.com.

165 In 1991, I wrote a story: Linda Villarosa, "Showdown at Sunrise," *Essence,* July 1991.

165 Nearly thirty years later: Linda Villarosa, "Pollution Is Killing Black Americans. This Community Fought Back," *New York Times Magazine,* July 28, 2020, www.nytimes.com.

165 Also in 1991, I wrote: Linda Villarosa, "Emergency: The Crisis in Our Health Care," *Essence,* Sept. 1991.

166 In 2016, while working: Cedric Sturdevant, interviews by author, Jackson, Miss., Oct. 4–9, 2016.

169 As I was working on the final draft: Sturdevant, phone interview by author, Jan. 26, 2017.

170 "Sometimes I wonder about that": Sturdevant, interview by author, Greenville, Miss., March 2, 2020.

170 An article published: Shreya Kangovi et al., "Evidence-Based Community Health Worker Program Addresses Unmet Social Needs and Generates Positive Return on Investment," *Health Affairs* 39, no. 2 (Feb. 2020), www.healthaffairs.org.

171 In 2010, the Affordable Care Act: MHP Salud, "History of Community Health Workers (CHWs) in America," accessed July 14, 2021, mhpsalud.org.

171 But our country of 331 million: U.S. Bureau of Labor Statistics, "Occupational Employment and Wages, May 2020: 21-1094 Community Health Workers," www.bls.gov.

171 countries like Ethiopia: USAID, "HRH2030 Assessment of Ethio-

pia's Health Extension Program Builds Evidence for Substantial Social Returns on HRH Investments," March 31, 2020, hrh2030program.org.

172 HEWs like Roba: World Bank, "Physicians (per 1000 People)," accessed July 14, 2021, data.worldbank.org.

172 "I never want someone": Aster Roba, interview by author, Ethiopia, Aug. 25, 2010.

172 The maternal mortality ratio: United Nations Population Fund, "Executive Summary, Trends in Maternal Mortality, 2000 to 2017," www.unfpa .org.

172 A 2020 report estimated: USAID, "HRH 2030 Assessment of Ethiopia's Health Extension Program," March 31, 2020, hrh2030program.org.

173 Additionally, a study that looked: Yibeltal Assefa et al., "Community Health Extension Program of Ethiopia, 2003–2018: Successes and Challenges Toward Universal Coverage for Primary Healthcare Services," *Globalization and Health* 15, no. 24 (2019), globalizationandhealth .biomedcentral.com.

173 Research from the World Health Organization: Zulfiqar A. Bhutta et al., "Global Experience of Community Health Workers for Delivery of Health Related Millennium Development Goals: A Systematic Review, Country Case Studies, and Recommendations for Integration into National Health Systems," Global Health Workforce Alliance, World Health Organization, accessed July 14, 2021, www.who.int.

173 The CHW concept: MHP Salud, "History of Community Health Workers (CHWs) in America."

173 A compilation of case studies: Henry B. Perry, "Health for the People: National Community Health Worker Programs from Afghanistan to Zimbabwe," Maternal and Child Survival Program, USAID, April 2020, pdf.usaid.gov.

174 A 2016 study published: Katy B. Kozhimannil et al., "Modeling the Cost-Effectiveness of Doula Care Associated with Reductions in Preterm Birth and Cesarean Delivery," *Birth* 1, no. 10 (Jan. 2016).

177 Louisiana has one of the highest rates: Centers for Disease Control and Prevention, "Infant Mortality Rates by State," accessed March 12, 2021, www.cdc.gov; Kaiser Family Foundation, "Infant Mortality Rate by Race/Ethnicity" (2018), www.kff.org.

177 highest rates of maternal mortality: Centers for Disease Control and Prevention, "Maternal Mortality by State, 2018," www.cdc.gov; Jia Benno et al., "Louisiana Pregnancy-Associated Mortality Review 2017 Report," Louisiana Department of Health (2020), ldh.la.gov.

177 Touro, a community hospital: Ryan Marx et al., "Touro Infirmary," *USA Today* (2019), www.usatoday.com.

178 In 2020, the American Medical Association: American Medical Association, "New AMA Policy Recognizes Racism as a Public Health Threat," Nov. 16, 2020, www.ama-assn.org.

178 an epidemiological review of research: Michael R. Kramer and Carol R. Hogue, "What Causes Racial Disparities in Very Preterm Birth? A Biosocial Perspective," *Epidemiologic Reviews* 31 (2009): 84–98.

178 "No one believes you": Carol Hogue, interview by author, Atlanta, Jan. 26, 2018.

179 One of the studies highlighted: Marion E. Gornick et al., "Effects of Race and Income on Mortality and Use of Services Among Medicare Beneficiaries," *New England Journal of Medicine,* Sept. 12, 1996, 791–99, www.nejm.org.

180 A 2020 study showed: Brad N. Greenwood et al., "Physician–Patient Racial Concordance and Disparities in Birthing Mortality for Newborns," *Proceedings of the National Academy of Sciences of the United States of America,* July 16, 2020.

180 In a widely circulated editorial: Mary T. Bassett, "#BlackLivesMatter—a Challenge to the Medical and Public Health Communities," *New England Journal of Medicine,* March 19, 2015, 1085–87, www.nejm.org.

180 Beginning in 2016: NYC Health, "Race to Justice," accessed July 14, 2021, www1.nyc.gov.

180 In that state, the rate of maternal deaths: California Maternal Quality Care Collaborative, "CA-PAMR (Maternal Mortality Review)," accessed July 14, 2021, www.cmqcc.org.

181 However, Black women did not benefit: California Maternal Quality Care Collaborative, "Birth Equity," accessed July 14, 2021, www.cmqcc.org.

181 she co-sponsored SB-464: California Legislative Information, "SB-464 California Dignity in Pregnancy and Childbirth Act (2019–2020)," leginfo.legislature.ca.gov.

181 In August 2018: Louisiana Department of Health, "Reducing Maternal Morbidity Initiative—Interim Report," accessed July 14, 2021, ldh.la.gov.

183 In the end, after twenty-one months: Louisiana Department of Health, "Reducing Maternal Morbidity Initiative—Final Report," updated May 25, 2021, ldh.la.gov.

184 The agency used the Undoing Racism model: Undoing Racism, People's Institute for Survival and Beyond, "How Can We Undo Racism," accessed July 14, 2021, pisab.org.

186 Even as the country grows more diverse: Association of American Medical Colleges, "Diversity in Medicine: Facts and Figures 2019," accessed July 14, 2021, www.aamc.org.

187 The much-cited 2016 University of Virginia study: Kelly M. Hoffman et al., "Racial Bias in Pain Assessment and Treatment Recommendations, and False Beliefs About Biological Differences Between Blacks and Whites," *Proceedings of the National Academy of Sciences of the United States of America* 113, no. 16 (2016): 4296–301, www.pnas.org.

187 Madeleine DeGrange: Madeleine DeGrange, Zoom interview by author, Sept. 21, 2020.

189 On a national level: White Coats for Black Lives, "How Does Your Medical School Add Up" (2021), whitecoats4blacklives.org.

189 In 2019, the group published: White Coats for Black Lives, "Racial Justice Report Card 2018," whitecoats4blacklives.org.

189 On the West Coast: Institute for Healing and Justice, accessed July 14, 2021, www.instituteforhealingandjustice.org.

190 In response, the multiracial student group: Noor Chadha et al., "Towards the Abolition of Biological Race in Medicine: Transforming Clinical Education, Research, and Practice," Institute for Healing and Justice in Medicine (2020), www.instituteforhealingandjustice.org.

190 In August 2020, a study: Darshali A. Vyas et al., "Hidden in Plain Sight—Reconsidering the Use of Race Correction in Clinical Algorithms," *New England Journal of Medicine,* Aug. 27, 2020, 874–82, www.nejm.org.

190 The Institute for Healing: Allison Inserro, "Flawed Racial Assumptions in eGFR Have Care Implications in CKD," *American Journal of Managed Care,* Oct. 25, 2020, www.ajmc.com.

191 In 2020, Naomi Nkinsi: Patricia Kullberg, "How Racism Gets Baked into Medical Decisions," *Science for the People,* Dec. 21, 2020, magazine .scienceforthepeople.org.

192 In September 2019, Stanley Goldfarb, MD: Stanley Goldfarb, "Take Two Aspirin and Call Me by My Pronouns," *Wall Street Journal,* Sept. 12, 2019, www.wsj.com.

192 Three days later, the *Journal's*: Editorial Board, "Corrupting Medical Education: The Reaction to Dr. Goldfarb's Op-Ed Proves His Point," *Wall Street Journal,* Sept. 15, 2019, www.wsj.com.

192 the *Journal* published another essay: Stanley Goldfarb, "Med School Needs an Overhaul," *Wall Street Journal,* April 13, 2020, www.wsj.com.

192 In March 2021, during a podcast: Apoorva Mandavilli, "Editor of JAMA Leaves After Outcry over Colleague's Remarks on Racism," *New York Times,* June 1, 2021, www.nytimes.com.

AFTERWORD

195 We would not be the first: Mary T. Bassett, "#BlackLivesMatter—a Challenge to the Medical and Public Health Communities," *New England Journal of Medicine,* March 19, 2015, 1085–87, www.nejm.org.

196 These talks, called "Something Inside": Hilary Beard, "Something Inside: Tools to Thrive: We Gonna Be Alright," Facebook, April 3, 2020, https:// www.facebook.com/hilarybeardauthor/videos/1037482676638919.

197 I was also reading notes: "The Spirit of 1848," Fall 1994; revised: Nov. 2000, Nov. 2001, March 2005, www.spiritof1848.org.

197 But the picture was becoming clear: Reis Thebault, Andrew Ba Tran, and Vanessa Williams, "The Coronavirus Is Infecting and Killing Black Americans at an Alarmingly High Rate," *Washington Post,* April 7, 2020, www.washingtonpost.com.

198 "There are so many stupid": Idris Elba (@idriselba), Twitter, March 16, 2020, 2:18 p.m., twitter.com/idriselba/status/1239617034901524481 ?lang=en.

198 On March 27: Senators Kamala D. Harris, Elizabeth Warren, and Cory A. Booker and Representatives Ayanna Pressley and Robin L. Kelly to Secretary Alex M. Azar II, March 27, 2020, www.warren.senate.gov.

198 Shortly after, the American Medical Association: American Medical Association, "Top Physician Orgs Urge COVID-19 Mortality Data by Race, Ethnicity," April 8, 2020, www.ama-assn.org.

198 The NAACP, Dr. Crear-Perry: We Must Count, "Disaggregate Covid-19 Data by Race, Genders, Socioeconomic Status," April 3, 2020, www .wemustcount.org.

199 While African Americans were 32 percent: Thebault, Tran, and Williams, "Coronavirus Is Infecting and Killing Black Americans at an Alarmingly High Rate."

201 "Baby, if you aren't feeling good": Nicole Charles, interview by author, New Orleans, April 7, 2020.

202 That day the Louisiana Department of Health: Chris McCrory, "COVID-19 Timeline: See How Fast Things Have Changed in Louisiana," WWL, March 22, 2020, www.wwltv.com.

203 At a news conference: "Louisiana Governor Edwards Coronavirus News Conference," C-SPAN, March 19, 2020, www.c-span.org.

203 guidelines the City of New Orleans: McCrory, "COVID-19 Timeline."

203 Dr. Maybank's op-ed ran: Aletha Maybank, "The Pandemic's Missing Data," *New York Times,* April 7, 2020, www.nytimes.com.

204 CDC released the first chunk: Shikha Garg et al., "Hospitalization Rates and Characteristics of Patients Hospitalized with Laboratory-Confirmed Coronavirus Disease 2019—COVID-NET, 14 States, March 1–30, 2020," *Morbidity and Mortality Weekly Report,* April 17, 2020, 458–64, www.cdc.gov.

204 Data from the Louisiana: Sheba Turk, "Racial Disparities in Louisiana's COVID-19 Death Rate Reflect Systemic Problems," WWL, April 7, 2020, www.wwltv.com.

204 "The coronavirus is very much under control": Kathryn Watson, "A Timeline of What Trump Has Said on Coronavirus," CBS News, April 3, 2020, www.cbsnews.com.

204 the president reiterated: Ibid.

204 The next day, an official: Megan Thielking and Helen Branswell, "CDC Expects 'Community Spread' of Coronavirus, as Top Official Warns Dis-

ruptions Could Be 'Severe,'" *Stat News,* Feb. 25, 2020, www.statnews .com.

204 "within a couple of days": Watson, "Timeline of What Trump Has Said on Coronavirus."

204 On March 9, the day: McCrory, "COVID-19 Timeline."

204 Trump compared the virus: Watson, "Timeline of What Trump Has Said on Coronavirus."

204 "The Fake News Media": Rebecca Klar, "Trump: 'Fake News Media,' Democrats Working to 'Inflame the CoronaVirus Situation,'" *Hill,* March 9, 2020, thehill.com.

205 Trump erroneously suggested: "President Trump claims injecting people with disinfectant could treat coronavirus," YouTube, April 24, 2020, www.youtube.com.

205 My story ran: Linda Villarosa, "'A Terrible Price': The Deadly Racial Disparities of Covid-19 in America," *New York Times Magazine,* May 3, 2020, updated Nov. 18, 2020, www.nytimes.com.

205 African Americans were more likely: Richard A. Oppel Jr. et al., "The Fullest Look Yet at the Racial Inequity of Coronavirus," *New York Times,* July 5, 2020, www.nytimes.com. The rates for Latinx and Native Americans were also elevated, especially as the pandemic progressed.

206 This pileup of deaths: Elizabeth Arias et al., "Provisional Life Expectancy Estimates for January Through June, 2020," Centers for Disease Control and Prevention, National Vital Statistics Systems, Report 010, Feb. 2021, www.cdc.gov.

206 An analysis of CDC data: Tiffany N. Ford, Sarah Reber, and Richard V. Reeves, "Race Gaps in COVID-19 Deaths Are Even Bigger Than They Appear," Brookings Institution, June 16, 2020, www.brookings.edu.

206 In an April radio interview: James Doubek, "Louisiana Sen. Cassidy Addresses Racial Disparities in Coronavirus Deaths," NPR, April 7, 2020, www.npr.org.

206 An article in *The Lancet:* Manish Pareek et al., "Ethnicity and COVID-19: An Urgent Public Health Research Priority," *Lancet,* April 21, 2020, www.thelancet.com.

206 Dr. Anthony Fauci: "COVID-19 Vaccine: Dr. Fauci Gets Why Black People Are Wary After Tuskegee Experiment," *BET News,* July 29, 2020, www.bet.com.

207 "communities of color . . . to step up": "White House Coronavirus News Conference," YouTube, April 10, 2020, www.youtube.com.

208 I watched a video: Jonathan Tilove, "Chanting 'Let Us Work!,' 'Fire Fauci!,' Protesters at Capitol Decry Virus Restrictions," *Statesman,* April 18, 2020, www.statesman.com.

209 Studies showed that white communities: Diana S. Grigsby-Toussaint et al., "Disparities in the Distribution of COVID-19 Testing Sites in

Black and Latino Areas in New York City," *Preventive Medicine* 147 (June 2021); Anuja Vaidya, "Most Rural US Counties Are in COVID-19 'Testing Deserts,' Analysis Finds," *Becker's Hospital Review,* June 23, 2020, www.beckershospitalreview.com.

209 As COVID rose: Nina Feldman, "The Black Doctors Working to Make Coronavirus Testing More Equitable," NPR, Oct. 1, 2020, www.npr.org.

209 A paper released: X. Wu et al., "Air Pollution and COVID-19 Mortality in the United States: Strengths and Limitations of an Ecological Regression Analysis," *Science Advances* 6, no. 45 (Nov. 2020).

210 With a nod toward: Centers for Disease Control and Prevention, "CDC COVID-19 Response Health Equity Strategy," updated Aug. 21, 2020, www.cdc.gov.

210 A study published: Michael W. Sjoding et al., "Racial Bias in Pulse Oximetry Measurement," *New England Journal of Medicine,* Dec. 17, 2020, 2477–78, www.nejm.org.

210 On December 4, she posted a video: Susan Moore, Facebook, Dec. 4, 2020, www.facebook.com/susan.moore.33671748/posts/3459157600869878.

211 Dr. Moore died two weeks later: John Eligon, "Black Doctor Dies of Covid-19 After Complaining of Racist Treatment," *New York Times,* Dec. 23, 2020, updated Dec. 25, 2020, www.nytimes.com.

211 An earlier statement: Dennis M. Murphy, "Directly Addressing the Issue of Racial Equity in Our Facilities," Indiana University Health, Dec. 24, 2020, iuhealth.org.

211 In Washington, D.C., 40 percent: Abby Goodnough and Jan Hoffman, "The Wealthy Are Taking an Outsize Share of Vaccines Meant for Poorer Neighborhoods," *New York Times,* Feb. 2, 2021, www.nytimes.com.

211 In December 2020, a poll: Liz Hamel et al., "KFF COVID-19 Vaccine Monitor: December 2020," Kaiser Family Foundation, Dec. 15, 2020, www.kff.org.

211 As with other medical studies: Samantha Artiga et al., "Racial Diversity Within COVID-19 Vaccine Clinical Trials: Key Questions and Answers," Kaiser Family Foundation, Jan. 26, 2021, www.kff.org.

212 Data compiled by the CDC: Centers for Disease Control and Prevention, "Overdose Deaths Accelerating During COVID-19," Dec. 17, 2020, www.cdc.gov.

212 "the most concerning in the United States": John Raby, "CDC: West Virginia HIV Wave Could Be 'Tip of the Iceberg,'" Associated Press, March 17, 2021, apnews.com.

212 in April 2021 he signed a bill: Cuneyt Dil, "West Virginia Lawmakers Approve Needle Exchange Regulations," Associated Press, April 10, 2021, apnews.com.

212 Nearly half of Black respondents: Yaphet Getachew et al., "Beyond the Case Count: The Wide-Ranging Disparities of COVID-19 in the United

States," Commonwealth Fund, Sept. 10, 2020, www.commonwealthfund
.org.

213 Nancy Krieger was interviewed: Isaac Chotiner, "The Interwoven
Threads of Inequality and Health," *New Yorker*, April 14, 2020, www
.newyorker.com.

213 In response to the ill-treatment: Aletha Maybank et al., "Say Her Name:
Dr. Susan Moore," *Washington Post*, Dec. 26, 2020, www.washingtonpost
.com.

213 Breonna Taylor, the Black medical worker: "Justice Denied: An Overview
of the Grand Jury Proceedings in the Breonna Taylor Case," NAACP
Legal Defense Fund, Oct. 27, 2020, www.naacpldf.org.

214 During the pandemic, California moved ahead: California Legislative
Information, "AB-241 Implicit Bias: Continuing Education: Requirements (2019–2020), October 10, 2019," leginfo.legislature.ca.gov.

214 His essay on Black Americans: Clyde W. Yancy, "COVID-19 and African Americans," *Journal of the American Medical Association* 323, no. 19
(2020): 1891–92, jamanetwork.com.

215 "COVID-19 has taken off the Band-Aid": Clyde Yancy, interview by
author, Chicago, April 18, 2020.

INDEX

A NOTE ABOUT THE AUTHOR

Linda Villarosa is a journalist in residence and an associate professor at the Craig Newmark Graduate School of Journalism at CUNY and also teaches journalism and Black studies at the City College of New York. She is a contributing writer to *The New York Times Magazine,* where she covers the intersection of race and health. Previously, she was an editor at *Essence* and a science editor at *The New York Times.*